Histopathological Stains and their Diagnostic Uses

Histopathological Stains and their Diagnostic Uses

JOHN D. BANCROFT
Senior Chief Technician, Department of Pathology,
University of Nottingham
and Part-time Course Tutor (Histopathology),
Trent Polytechnic, Nottingham

ALAN STEVENS, MB, BS, MRCPath.
Senior Lecturer in Pathology, Department of Pathology,
University of Nottingham
and Honorary Consultant Pathologist,
Trent Health Authority

Photography by

W. H. BRACKENBURY,
Department of Pathology,
University of Nottingham

Foreword by

Professor I. M. P. DAWSON, MA, MD, FRCP, FRCPath.
Department of Pathology,
University of Nottingham

CHURCHILL LIVINGSTONE
EDINBURGH LONDON AND NEW YORK 1975

CHURCHILL LIVINGSTONE
Medical Division of Longman Group Limited

Distributed in the United States of America by
Longman Inc., New York and by associated
companies, branches and representatives throughout
the world.

ISBN 0 443 01226 1

Library of Congress Catolog Card Number 74–81753

Printed in Great Britain

Foreword

Techniques in histopathology and histochemistry are often likened to those in cookery, with the implication that a successful result is largely unscientific and anyway depends more on the cook than the recipe. Cookery books, however, have become far more scientific over the years, as anyone selecting a wifely birthday present soon discovers; the same cannot be said for many manuals on histological and histochemical methodology, which still very much tend to present their techniques on an 'ours not to reason why', take it or leave it basis. The reader of this short book will find a refreshing change, for a genuine attempt is made to explain the basis on which staining reactions are performed, so that one can make an intelligent choice of techniques for each particular purpose, and have at least some idea of why different dyes delineate different substances, and how far a positive 'stain' reflects an underlying chemical structure. Apart from raising the standard of reporting on histological material, such knowledge immensely enhances the interest. It also serves to draw together technician and pathologist, for the best cooperation in any field occurs when all understand the reason for what they are doing; the fact that this book results from such a cooperation, reflecting as it were the production and consumer interests is one of its strengths.

I can well remember as a junior searching book after book not for details of how to prepare tissue, which was well drummed into us, but of why I did what I did; this book would have saved me a deal of trouble. I warmly wish it well and look forward to possessing my copy.

Nottingham, 1974   I. M. P. DAWSON

Preface

Our aims are that this short book will serve a dual purpose. First, it is an attempt to explain simply to practising and to trainee pathologists the underlying principles of common histological stains and relevant histochemical methods, and their applications in diagnostic histopathology. Secondly, it is aimed at histopathology technologists who, all too often, work in a vacuum, performing staining techniques without understanding the indications for them. From the pathologist's point of view most textbooks of histopathological techniques are too long and detailed, and for technologists these same books are lacking in clinical relevance. We have striven therefore to produce a book which is sufficiently non-technical to inform the pathologist, and yet to contain enough clinical information to interest the technologist.

We consider this book a useful preparation for the Advanced Final Examination in Histopathology of the Institute of Medical Laboratory Technology, and for the Higher National Certificate in Medical Laboratory Science (Histopathology). It should also prove a useful adjunct for pathologists studying for the Primary and Final Examinations for Membership of the Royal College of Pathologists (MRCPath). We have included at the end of some chapters a short list of relevant further reading, for both technologist and pathologist.

J.D.B.
A.S.

Nottingham, 1974

Acknowledgements

The authors wish to express their gratitude to their families and colleagues for their forbearance during the preparation of this book, and especially to Professor I. M. P. Dawson for his encouragement, interest and tolerance. We owe a special vote of thanks to Mr Paul Bradbury and Mr Keith Gordon of the Pathology Department, City Hospital, Nottingham, who read the entire manuscript and offered many helpful suggestions and criticisms. Our thanks are also expressed to Professor I. M. P. Dawson, Dr G. Stirling and Dr G. Robinson of the Department of Pathology, University of Nottingham, and to Mr H. C. Cook of the West Middlesex Hospital, all of whom read and criticised various chapters.

One of us (A. S.) wishes to take this opportunity of thanking Mr Jim Willder, Chief Technician in the Department of Pathology, Guy's Hospital, for initiating and stimulating his interest in histopathological staining.

Finally we thank Miss Colleen Peel for her speedy and impeccable typing of the manuscript and Mr Bill Brackenbury, whose photographic skills often made silk purses out of sows' ears.

Contents

CHAPTER 1

Haematoxylin and Eosin and the Applications of Haematoxylins

This is a natural dye that is obtained from the heartwood of the tree *Haematoxylin campechianum*. It is a native of the Mexican state of Campeche after which the tree is named, but it is now mainly cultivated in the West Indies. The trees when felled are stripped of bark and sapwood and the heartwood exported as logwood. Haematoxylin is extracted from the logwood with hot water and precipitated out in the presence of urea (Lamb, 1974). Since 1840 it has become the most used and adaptable histological stain, despite its poor staining qualities when used alone. To obtain a suitable staining solution with haematoxylin, two conditions must be fulfilled; first, its active constituent, haematein, must be produced; secondly, the stain must be used with a mordant. In alum haematoxylins the mordant is incorporated in the staining solution, usually potassium aluminium sulphate. In iron haematoxylins the mordant is a ferric salt (usually ferric chloride or ferric ammonium sulphate), and is often used prior to the dye.

Haematein is produced by the oxidation of haematoxylin. This is brought about by the use of chemical oxidising agents, e.g. sodium iodate, or by the traditional method of exposure to light and air, termed 'ripening'. The instant ripening by using oxidising agents gives good results and sodium iodate is very satisfactory for this purpose. Oxidation by exposure takes up to 15 weeks.

Haematoxylins are divided into two groups:

(a) *alum haematoxylins* which utilise aluminium ions (potassium alum, etc.). Examples include Mayer's, Ehrlich's, Harris's and Cole's haematoxylins.

(b) *iron haematoxylins* which employ ferric ions (ferric ammonium sulphate and ferric chloride), examples being Heidenhain's and Weigert's haematoxylins.

Alum haematoxylins

A considerable number of alum haematoxylins are cited in the literature, each worker having his own preference. In the U.K. the five most popular are probably Mayer's, Harris's, Cole's, Ehrlich's and Delafield's variants. These haematoxylins are usually used in routine haematoxylin and eosin stains. The acidified solutions of Ehrlich's and Mayer's are particularly suitable, for at a more acid pH they have greater affinity for the nuclei and will stain other tissue components less.

The first alum haematoxylin was that of Böhmer (1865) and most of the existing solutions are a modification of his original formula. The staining time of alum haematoxylins will vary for many reasons, one of which is the amount of oxidation the haematoxylin has undergone. This is of prime importance, for it governs the amount of haematein in the staining solution and consequently the strength of the stain. Other factors that play an important part in the staining time are the number of sections already stained, the fixative employed, and whether or not the tissue has been subjected to prolonged treatment with acid solutions, as in decalcification. In some instances the staining time will be considerably increased; times of 5 to 30 minutes are usual, depending upon which stain is used, the strength of the stain and the type of section to be stained.

A major drawback of the alum haematoxylins is their lack of resistance to dyes in acid solutions (e.g. van Gieson). A section overstained in Mayer's haemalum and then treated with van Gieson will appear with a very pale nuclear stain when viewed under the microscope. For this reason it is advisable when working with acid solutions to use iron haematoxylins or, as an alternative, the celestin blue-alum haematoxylin technique.

Celestin blue

This dye was first suggested by Proescher and Arkush (1928) as a nuclear stain, and was further explored by Lendrum (1935) who stated that the resistance of celestin blue to the action of acid allows its use in van Gieson's stain. Lendrum and McFarlane (1940) advised the use of celestin blue as a mordant to alum haematoxylin. The ferric salts in the celestin blue solution, in combination with Mayer's haematoxylin, give a strong nuclear stain that is reasonably resistant to acid dye solutions.

The combination of celestin blue and Mayer's or Cole's haematoxylin has become a feature of staining techniques which employ a nuclear stain followed by an acid solution (e.g. van Gieson, and the multiple connective tissue stains). To a large extent this procedure has replaced the iron haematoxylin technique, being easier to use and eliminating the need for an additional haematoxylin solution.

Iron haematoxylins

This alternative to the alum haematoxylins was first produced by Benda (1886); today two iron haematoxylins are standard, Weigert's (1904) and Heidenhain's (1892, 1896). In these stains ferric salts are used both as oxidising agents and mordants: the salts used are ferric chloride and ferric sulphate. Great care has to be taken with these solutions to see that over-oxidation does not occur. For this reason iron haematoxylins are kept as two solutions, mordant and stain. In the case of Weigert's stain they are mixed before use; for Heidenhain's they are used consecutively.

APPLICATIONS

The use of iron haematoxylins as nuclear stains has lessened in recent years with the increase in popularity of the celestin blue-alum haematoxylin technique.

Heidenhain's iron haematoxylin is used as a *regressive* stain and needs careful differentiation under microscopic control. It is used to demonstrate muscle striations (Fig. 1.1), myelin, mitochondria, chromatin and chromosomes. *Weigert's iron haematoxylin* is normally used as a nuclear stain; it is a *progressive* stain and once the correct staining time has been established for a particular batch of stain no differentiation is required.

Haematoxylin and eosin

This is the routine staining method used in all types of histology laboratories.

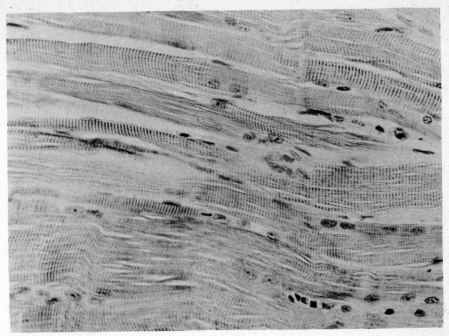

Figure 1.1 Normal striated muscle stained by Heidenhain's haematoxylin method. After accurate differentiation the striations are elegantly demonstrated. Magnification (× 392)

One of the first skills required of a technologist is to be able to produce high quality results with this stain. A good H & E stain will demonstrate a number of structures including cell nuclei, red blood cells, cytoplasm and some connective tissues. To attain this, the correct haematoxylin must be used to stain the nuclei, and then accurately differentiated so as to leave no excess stain in the background.

A section properly stained with eosin will demonstrate structures in various shades of red and pink. Sections need to be overstained with eosin, well differentiated in running tap water, slowly dehydrated through graded alcohols, cleared in xylol and mounted in a resinous medium.

Mallory's phosphotungstic acid haematoxylin (PTAH)

This haematoxylin, now used to demonstrate many tissue elements, was originally described (Mallory, 1897, 1900) to show fibrin, striated muscle fibres and neuroglia, using a 1 per cent aqueous phosphotungstic acid solution. Modifications in common use utilise a 2 per cent phosphotungstic acid solution. The best results are obtained with a staining solution prepared by mixing unripened haematoxylin and the phosphotungstic acid solution, and then allowing natural ripening in sunlight. Unfortunately this takes several months, but when ripe the stain will last for several years. Two methods are available to avoid this long ripening period. First, haematein may be used instead of haematoxylin, removing the need for oxidation of the haematoxylin; the solution is ready for use after two days. Secondly, potassium permanganate may be used as an oxidising agent for the haematoxylin, but this produces an unstable staining solution which does not reach peak staining ability for about seven days, (although it may be used during this time). Its shelf life is restricted because it deteriorates quicker than the other two types of stain. Phosphotungstic acid haematoxylin is used as a progressive stain, although some degree of differentiation can be obtained with experience during the dehydration stage. Many laboratories use a Mallory bleach (acidified potassium permanganate followed by oxalic acid) which is said to aid differential staining, whilst others prefer to use 4 per cent iron alum as a mordant. In our hands both methods work satisfactorily but we use the former for routine purposes. Most fixatives give satisfactory results with this method, Zenker giving particularly good results.

The haematoxylins are summarised in Table 1.1.

Table 1.1. Summary of haematoxylins and their uses

Haematoxylin	Type	Use with celestin blue	Main application
Mayer's	Alum	Yes	General use and bone
Harris's	Alum	Yes	Sharp nuclear staining. Cytology
Cole's	Alum	Yes	General use
Ehrlich's	Alum	No	General use, mucins and bone
Weigert's	Iron	–	Nuclei with acid counterstains, e.g. van Gieson
Heidenhain's	Iron	–	Muscle striations, myelin, chromatin, mitochondria, etc.
Mallory's PTAH	Phosphotungstic	–	Collagen, muscle, fibrin, neuroglia fibres, etc

FORMULATION OF SOME COMMON HAEMATOXYLIN SOLUTIONS

Mayer's haematoxylin (Mayer, 1903)

This is an example of an alum haematoxylin, artificially ripened with sodium iodate.

Haematoxylin	1 g
Distilled water	1000 ml
Potassium alum	50 g
Citric acid	1 g
Chloral hydrate	50 g
Sodium iodate	200 mg

Warm the distilled water, and dissolve the haematoxylin, potassium alum and sodium iodate in it. Stir until all the potassium alum is dissolved. Then add the chloral and citric acid. Bring the solution to the boil and allow to boil for 5 minutes. Cool, filter and leave overnight before use. Staining time 10–20 minutes.

Mayer's haematoxylin (modified for bone sections)

Solution 1

Haematoxylin	2 g
Absolute alcohol	40 ml

Solution 2

Potassium alum	100 g
Distilled water	600 ml

Heat slightly to help the alum to dissolve. Mix solutions 1 and 2 and boil for 2 minutes. Make up to 2000 ml with distilled water and add 400 mg sodium iodate. Staining time for bone sections 40–60 minutes.

Harris's haematoxylin (Harris, 1900)

This is an alum haematoxylin, chemically ripened with mercuric oxide.

Haematoxylin	2.5 g
Absolute alcohol	25 ml
Potassium alum	50 g
Distilled water	500 ml
Mercuric oxide	1.25 g
Glacial acetic acid	20 ml

Dissolve the haematoxylin in the absolute alcohol and add to the alum previously dissolved in the warm distilled water in a two-litre flask. Rapidly bring the solution to the boil. While the stain is boiling add the mercuric oxide, then plunge the flask into cold water. When the solution is cold add the acetic acid. Staining time 5–10 minutes.

Ehrlich's haematoxylin (Ehrlich, 1886)

Haematoxylin	2 g
Absolute alcohol	100 ml
Glycerin	100 ml
Distilled water	100 ml
Glacial acetic acid	10 ml
Potassium alum	15 g approx.

The haematoxylin is dissolved in the alcohol, followed by the other chemicals. Best results are obtained by allowing the stain to ripen by exposure to sun and light; this will take about 8 weeks. Sodium iodate (300 mg) may be added to the solution to oxidise the haematoxylin and render it ready for use immediately. Staining time 20 minutes.

Celestin blue

Celestin blue B	2.5 g
Ferric ammonium sulphate	25 g
Glycerin	70 ml
Distilled water	500 ml

For use with Mayer's or Cole's haematoxylins.

Weigert's iron haematoxylin

Solution A

Haematoxylin	1 g
Absolute alcohol	100 ml

Solution B

30 per cent aqueous ferric chloride (anhydrous)	4 ml
Hydrochloric acid (concentrated)	1 ml
Distilled water	95 ml

Equal parts of A and B are mixed immediately before use. Solution B should be added to solution A. The staining solution should be a violet-black colour. If it is brown it should be discarded. Staining time 30 minutes.

Heidenhain's iron haematoxylin

Solution A

Ferric ammonium sulphate	5 g
Distilled water	100 ml

It is important that only the clear violet crystals are used.

Solution B

Haematoxylin	0.5 g
Absolute alcohol	10 ml
Distilled water	90 ml

Dissolve the haematoxylin in the alcohol then add water. Average staining time 1 hour in each solution.

PTAH solution

Using haematein

Haematein	0.5 g
Phosphotungstic acid	5.0 g
Distilled water	500 ml

Dissolve the haematein in 100 ml of distilled water, then dissolve the phosphotungstic acid in the other 400 ml and mix. Store in an airtight reagent bottle; ready to use next day.

Self ripening stain

Haematoxylin	0.5 g
Phosphotungstic acid	5.0 g
Distilled water	500 ml

Ripening will take several months.

Chemically ripened

Haematoxylin	0.5 g
Phosphotungstic acid	10.0 g
Distilled water	500 ml
0.25 per cent aqueous potassium permanganate	25 ml

Dissolve the haematoxylin in 100 ml of the distilled water, then dissolve the phosphotungstic acid in the other 400 ml. Mix the two solutions and add the potassium permanganate. The solution is ready for use next day.

STAINING METHODS

Haematoxylin and eosin stain for routine use

SOLUTIONS
Haematoxylin
  See pages 4, 5.

Eosin

Eosin	10 g
Distilled water	1000 ml

0.5 ml acetic acid may be added to the above solution to sharpen the staining. Moulds will grow but these are harmless and can be filtered off, or thymol may be added to the solution.

METHOD
1. Dewax sections in xylol, then treat with graded alcohols and place in water.
2. Remove fixation pigments if necessary.
3. Stain in haematoxylin of choice for 5–20 minutes.
4. Wash well in running tap water till sections go a darker blue, 5 minutes.
5. Remove background staining and excess stain by differentiating in 1 per cent acid alcohol (1 per cent HCl in 70 per cent alcohol) for 5–10 seconds.
6. Wash well in tap water until sections regain blue colour, 5 minutes.
7. Stain in 1 per cent eosin for 10 minutes.
8. Wash in running tap water for 5 minutes.
9. Dehydrate slowly through graded alcohols to xylol.
10. Mount in DPX.

RESULTS
Nuclei: *blue-black.*
Cytoplasm: *different shades of pink.*
Muscle fibres: *deep pink.*
Collagen: *light pink.*
Red blood cells: *orange red.*

NOTES
1. Sections are overstained with haematoxylin. The excess stain is removed by treatment with acid alcohol. The section is checked microscopically

until the background is clear and the nuclei well stained.

2. The 'blueing' stage involves placing the sections after treatment with acid alcohol into alkaline tap water. In some laboratories the tap water is not alkaline enough to produce this 'blueing' rapidly enough, in which case Scott's tap water substitute should be used (see p. 31).

3. Mayer's, Harris's and Ehrlich's haematoxylins give the best results in our hands; Ehrlich's and the modified Mayer's (p. 5) are ideal for bone sections.

Heidenhain's iron haematoxylin

SOLUTIONS
   See page 6.

METHOD
   This haematoxylin is capable of staining many structures. Staining is regressive and requires skilful differentiation. Sections $3–5\,\mu$ should be used.

1. Place sections in xylol, then down to water.
2. Place in mordant in 5 per cent ferric ammonium sulphate in distilled water for 1 hour.
3. Rinse in distilled water.
4. Stain in haematoxylin solution for 1 hour (see p. 6).
5. Wash in running tap water.
6. Differentiate in the mordant solution or the mordant solution diluted 50:50 with distilled water until required structures are visible. Alternate a rinse in the differentiator with a rinse in tap water.
7. Wash in running tap water for 10 minutes.
8. Dehydrate through graded alcohols to xylene, clear and mount in DPX.

RESULTS
Mitochondria, muscle striations, myelin, etc.: *black-grey*.

NOTES
1. The time needed in mordant and stain varies according to the fixative used; times of up to 12 hours may be required. Formalin and formol sublimate usually require 1 hour. The time in mordant and stain should be the same.
2. Differentiation requires practice, using the microscope to check the stain after each dip into the differentiator followed by the rinse in water.

PTAH

SOLUTIONS
Postchromate solution

10 per cent hydrochloric acid in methylated spirit	12 ml
3 per cent aqueous potassium dichromate	36 ml

Acidified potassium permanganate

0.5 per cent aqueous potassium permanganate	50 ml
3.0 per cent sulphuric acid	2.5 ml

PTAH solution
See page 6.

METHOD
1. Place sections in xylol, then down to water.
2. Place in postchromate solution for 30 minutes.
3. Wash in tap water.
4. Treat with acid permanganate solution for 1 minute.
5. Wash in tap water.
6. Bleach in 1 per cent oxalic acid.
7. Rinse in tap water.
8. Transfer to Mallory's PTAH solution overnight.
9. Dehydrate through graded alcohols.
10. Clear in xylene and mount in DPX.

RESULTS
Muscle: *dark blue*.
Neuroglia fibres: *dark blue*.
Fibrin: *dark blue*.
Nuclei: *light blue*.
Collagen: *rose red*.
Bone: *rose red*.

NOTES
1. In place of the postchroming and 'Mallory bleach', sections may be mordanted with 4 per cent iron alum for 30 minutes.
2. Dehydration must be rapid, as water and alcohols remove the staining.
3. Staining is progressive.

REFERENCES

BENDA, C. (1886). Uber eine neue Farbemethode der centralnervensystems, und theoretisches uber Haematoxylinfarbungen. *Arch. Anat. physiol. Anat. abt. physiol. abt.*, 562.

BOHMER, F. (1865). Zur pathologischen Anatomie de meningitis cerbromedullaris epidemica. *Aertzl intelligenz Munich*, **12**, 539.

COLE, E. C. (1943). Studies on hematoxylin stains. *Stain Technol.*, **18**, 125.

EHRLICH, P. (1886). Fragekasten. *Z. wiss. Mikr.*, **3**, 150.

HEIDENHAIN, M. (1892). *Ueber Kern und Protoplasma*. Leipzig: Kolliker.

HEIDENHAIN, M. (1896). Noch einmal uber die Darstellung der Centralkorper durch Eisenhamatoxylin nebst einigen allgemeinen bemerkungen uber die Hamatoxylinfarben. *Z. wiss. Mikr.*, **13**, 186.

HARRIS, H. F. (1900). On the rapid conversion of haematoxylin into haematein in staining reactions. *J. appl. Microsc. lab. Meth.*, **3**, 777.

LAMB, R. A. (1974). Personal communication.

LENDRUM, A. C. (1935). Celestin blue as a nuclear stain. *J. Path. Bact.*, **40**, 75.

LENDRUM, A. C. & McFARLANE, D. (1940). A controllable modification of Mallory's trichrome staining method. *J. Path. Bact.*, **50**, 381.

MALLORY, F. B. (1897). On certain improvements in histological technique (PTAH). *J. exp. Med.*, **2**, 529.

MALLORY. F. B. (1900). A contribution to staining methods. *J. exp. Med.*, **5**, 15.

MAYER, P. (1903). Notiz uber hamatein und hamalaun. *Z. wiss. Mikr.*, **20**, 409.

PROESCHER, F. & ARKUSH, A. S. (1928). Metallic lakes of the oxasines (Gallamin blue, Gallocyanin and Coelestin blue) as nuclear stain substitutes for hematoxylin. *Stain Technol.*, **3**, 28.

WEIGERT, K. (1904). Eine Kleine Verbesserung der hamatoxylin van Gieson methode. *Z. wiss. Mikr.*, **21**, 1.

CHAPTER 2

Carbohydrates and the Periodic Acid Schiff Reaction

The terminology of carbohydrates is difficult to follow, partly because over the years many terms have come into use which are not strictly accurate; in addition there is often more than one term for the same substance. The classification of carbohydrates is an incredibly complex matter and has become increasingly so in recent years with additional staining procedures and the identification of more substances. Few of the carbohydrates identified by biochemical methods can be demonstrated positively in tissue sections by the histochemical techniques available at present. A classification of carbohydrates by histochemical reactions cannot be compared to a biochemically based classification, due to the lack of specific chemical information forthcoming from the histochemical reaction. A new terminology for a histochemical classification was suggested by Spicer, Leppi and Stoward (1965). The following classification is based on that paper and the writings of Meyer (1966), Pearse (1968) and Cook (1972).

CLASSIFICATION OF CARBOHYDRATES

The carbohydrates are divided into three groups: polysaccharides (e.g. glycogen), neutral mucosubstances (e.g. neutral glycoproteins) and acid mucosubstances (e.g. epithelial sialomucins).

Polysaccharides

Glycogen is the only polysaccharide normally demonstrated in animal tissue sections by histochemical means. Other members of the group include cellulose and starch which are found in plants, and chitin in invertebrates and plants.

GLYCOGEN

Glycogen is an important storage carbohydrate in man, and as such is found in the hepatocytes in the liver. It is a vital substance in the production of energy, and is therefore also present in skeletal and cardiac muscle. Chemically glycogen is a polymer composed of units of D-glucose, and spontaneous breakdown of glycogen to glucose occurs very rapidly after death of the tissue; it is imperative therefore to obtain rapid and adequate fixation of any tissue in which glycogen is to be demonstrated, but if this is not possible, small pieces of tissue may be refrigerated for not longer than 24 hours before fixation.

A great deal has been written about fixation techniques for glycogen, especially in regard to its solubility in water. It has become clear in recent years that many of the earlier statements were over-cautious. Originally, tissue to be used for the demonstration of glycogen was fixed in absolute alcohol to avoid loss due to solubility in water. Alcohol, however, causes severe shrinkage

11

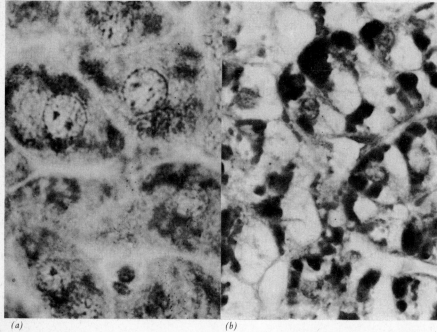

(a)   (b)

Figure 2.1 (a) Liver stained by the PAS reaction to show the distribution of glycogen within the liver parenchyma. The section has been prepared by a freeze-drying method which is particularly suitable for the accurate demonstration of polysaccharides. PAS (× 1360)

(b) Liver stained by the PAS reaction to show glycogen in a section prepared in the normal manner; note that the stainable glycogen appears to be congregated in the cytoplasm at one side of the cell only. This effect is called 'streaming artefact'. PAS (× 1120)

and penetrates poorly into tissue and should be avoided as a fixative on its own. During fixation, glycogen becomes insoluble and the classical streaming artefact is produced as the fixative penetrates the block of tissue (Fig. 2.1).

Routine fixation with formol saline will give acceptable results, but Lillie's AAF and Gendre's fixative give the best results in the authors' experience (see Appendix 1).

Neutral mucosubstances

These contain sugars and do not contain any free acidic groups or sulphate esters. They are found in the lining epithelium of the stomach, Brunner's glands of the duodenum and the colonic goblet cells (Cook, 1972). They fail to stain with any of the mucosubstance stains, with the exception of the periodic acid Schiff (PAS) reaction.

Acid mucosubstances

The acid mucosubstances can be subdivided into sulphated and non-sulphated types.

SULPHATED MUCOSUBSTANCES

These are divided into two types:
(a) Connective tissue mucosubstances (acidic, strongly sulphated).
(b) Epithelial mucosubstances (acidic, weakly sulphated).

Connective tissue mucosubstances

This group can be divided into two subdivisions; i.e. those containing hyaluronosulphate (as found in the cornea), heparan sulphate and keratan sulphate, and a second group which contains chondroitin sulphates A and B and mixtures of A and B. These are found in heart valves, aorta, skin and cartilage. They give weak or negative staining reactions with alcian blue at pH 2.5 but a moderate result at pH 0.5. They are metachromatic with azure 'A' at pH 2.0 and negative with the PAS reaction.

Epithelial mucosubstances

These contain sulphate esters which react differently from those described above. The epithelial mucosubstances are found in submandibular salivary glands, duodenal and colonic goblet cells (Cook, 1972). They differ from the strongly sulphated connective tissue mucosubstances in that they give a weak PAS reaction and a positive result with alcian blue at pH 2.5. They are strongly metachromatic with azure 'A' at pH 2.0.

NON-SULPHATED MUCOSUBSTANCES

These are divided into two types.
(a) Sialic acid rich (acidic, non–sulphated).
(b) Hexuronic acid rich (acidic, non–sulphated).

Sialic acid rich
(a) Connective tissue mucosubstances.
(b) Epithelial mucosubstances.

These mucosubstances contain sialic acid which is a derivative of neuraminic acid. The reactive groups are carboxyl groups. They contain no sulphate esters and are found in the goblet cells of lung and intestine and also in salivary glands. They stain with alcian blue at pH 2.5 and are metachromatic at pH 3.0 and above with azure 'A'. They also give a positive result with the PAS reaction.

Note that the existence of connective tissue sialic acid rich, non–sulphated mucosubstances ('connective tissue sialomucins') is disputed by some authorities; the proponents believe that they occur in cartilage.

Hexuronic acid rich

The mucosubstances present in this group contain hyaluronic acid. They have carboxyl groups as the reactive groups. These mucosubstances are found in umbilical cord, synovium, mesothelial cells and skin. The staining reactions are similar to the above group with the exception of the PAS reaction which is negative. The malignant tumour of pleural mesothelium, the mesothelioma, produces excessive amounts of hexuronic acid rich, non–sulphated acidic mucosubstances.

Other carbohydrates

MUCOPROTEINS

These are complex substances which consist of polysaccharide in chemical combination with protein. The term mucoprotein covers substances that contain more than 4 per cent carbohydrate whereas glycoproteins have less than 4 per cent. Mucoproteins are found in basement membranes and in the mucoid cells of the pituitary. They are demonstrated by the PAS reaction.

MUCOLIPIDS

As the title suggests these substances contain polysaccharides and lipid (in the form of fatty acid complexes). In some instances sialic acid is also in combination. The PAS reaction will usually give a positive reaction for mucolipids. Examples of mucolipids include the cerebrosides and gangliosides, found in large amounts in the brain and other organs in the group of disorders known as the 'lipid storage diseases' (see Chap. 3).

DEMONSTRATION OF MUCOSUBSTANCES

A large number of staining methods exist to demonstrate the many muco-substances. Many of the more recent methods which help to classify the individual substances are beyond the scope of this book, but should be followed by pathologist and technologist with interest, along with the use of blocking, methylation, saponification and enzyme digestion techniques. This is the only way that the complicated subject of carbohydrates can be unravelled histochemically. The main reactions are considered below.

Alcian blue

This is the best available routine method to demonstrate acidic weakly sulphated or acidic non-sulphated mucosubstances, when used at pH 3.0. Above pH 3 the specificity for acid mucosubstances disappears. Much work has been carried out in regard to the specificity of alcian blue. Scott and Dorling (1965), using alcian blue in varying electrolyte solutions, were able to show the different types of acid mucosubstances by altering the molarity of the electrolyte (magnesium chloride) added to the alcian blue stain. This concept (known as the 'critical electrolyte concentration') has done much to improve our knowledge of acid mucosubstances. However, it must be admitted that the validity of the concept has been disputed on theoretical grounds (Goldstein and Horobin, 1974). The use of alcian blue with different molarities of electrolyte solutions, and the use of different pH levels (see Table 2.2, p. 16), allows for the demonstration of many separate mucosubstances.

Metachromasia

The majority of acid mucosubstances will give a positive result with either toluidine blue, azure A or thionin. As with alcian blue, the varying of pH will help with the further identification of the substance. Metachromatic staining below pH 3.0 is usually due to *acidic sulphated mucosubstances*. Above pH 3.5 only the acidic non-sulphated mucosubstances give the characteristic pink staining (Spicer, 1960).

Mucicarmine

This popular empirical method has long been used to demonstrate muco-substances. In our hands it stains well only the acidic weakly sulphated muco-substances, the sialic acid rich, and hexuronic acid rich, non-sulphated mucosubstances, whilst being unreliable with other mucosubstances.

PAS reaction

This method gives controversial results with acidic mucosubstances. It is accepted that some of the sialic acid rich, non-sulphated mucosubstances, (especially the epithelial sialomucins) will give a positive result, while the acidic sulphated mucosubstances usually give a negative result.

THE PERIODIC ACID SCHIFF REACTION

This technique is bound up with the whole of carbohydrate histochemistry. It is used to demonstrate many carbohydrate-containing structures (e.g. fungi). The principle of the reaction is the production of dialdehydes in the carbohydrate-containing substances by oxidation with periodic acid, and the subsequent combination of the aldehydes with Schiff's reagent to give a substituted dye which is red in colour, and localised at the site of the aldehydes. A summary of PAS-positive material is given in Table 2.1.

Table 2.1. PAS positive material

Material	Example	Result	Alternative staining method
Polysaccharide	Glycogen	Strong	Best's carmine
Neutral mucosubstances	Colonic goblet cells	Strong	–
(Some) acid mucosubstances	Acidic non-sulphated, sialic acid-containing	Moderate	Alcian blue
Basement membranes	Glomerular basement membrane kidney	Moderate	Methenamine silver
Pigments	Lipofuscin	Moderate	Long ZN
Lipids	Cerebrosides	Moderate	–
Amyloid (some deposits only)	–	Weak	Congo red
Cartilage	–	Strong	Toluidine blue
Fungi	Candida	Moderate	Methenamine silver
Pituitary	Mucoid cells	Strong	Trichrome

Oxidation

Periodic acid was used as an oxidising agent by Malaprade (1934) for the chemical estimation of glycols. It was also used as a reagent for polysaccharides by Jackson and Hudson (1937). In histochemistry it was first used by McManus (1948) for demonstrating mucin, then further work by Lillie (1947a, b) and Hotchkiss (1948) enabled the PAS reaction to be used to identify glycogen and some mucosubstances in tissue sections. Periodic acid will break double carbon bonds in various structures where they are present as $1:2$ glycol groups (CHOH—CHOH) converting them into dialdehyde (CHO—CHO). The equivalent amino or alkylamino derivatives are also converted into dialdehydes. The important property of the periodic acid, which renders it immeasurably superior to other oxidising agents, is that under the histochemical conditions used, it will *not* further oxidise the resulting aldehydes. As a result, the accuracy and standardisation are considerably easier. Periodic acid can be used at any strength between 0.5 per cent and 2.5 per cent without much appreciable difference though 1 per cent is commonly used. Originally

Hotchkiss used alcohol as the solvent for periodic acid as it was thought at that time that the polysaccharide or its reaction product would be soluble in water. The use of 70 per cent alcohol as a solvent requires an extension of the 10 minutes oxidation time with periodic acid, as well as producing a less intense colour reaction. Pearse (1968) states that temperature is an important factor with the use of periodic acid; at temperatures above normal room temperature non-specific oxidation will occur. If the temperature is elevated then the aldehydes will be further oxidised to carboxylic acids, and groups other than the specific 1:2 glycol groups may be oxidised. The following three factors should be observed when using periodic acid as an oxidising agent:

(a) oxidation time to be limited to 10 minutes.
(b) oxidation should not be carried out at a higher temperature than 20°C.
(c) periodic acid solution should be pH 3–5·0.

Prepared solutions of the 1 per cent periodic acid should be kept in the refrigerator and may be used at any temperature between 4°C and 20°C. Under normal conditions a 1 per cent solution of periodic acid will give the correct pH range (Table 2.2).

Table 2.2. Staining of mucosubstances at various pH levels

Stain	pH	Strong positively
Alcian blue	2.5	Acidic non-sulphated (both types) Acidic sulphated (epithelial only)
Alcian blue	0.5	Acidic sulphated (connective tissue type only)
Azure A/Tol. blue	2.0	Acidic sulphated (both epithelial and connective tissue types)
Azure A/Tol. blue	6.0	Acidic non-sulphated (both types)
PAS	5.0	Neutral mucosubstances; acidic non-sulphated (containing sialic acid only) Glycolipids, mucolipids

Schiff's reagent

This solution was first described for biochemical work by Schiff. There are many variations of the original formula and all the accepted ones give good results. When basic fuchsin is treated with sulphurous acid, a colourless product is produced, known as Schiff's reagent. Basic fuchsin is a mixture of pararosaniline, magenta II and other compounds. Pararosaniline is the principal consistuent of basic fuchsin and is usually present as an acetate or chloride. Due to its quinoid structure the dye is relatively unstable, and when treated with sulphurous acid it produces N-aminosulphinic acid (Schiff's reagent). This solution, when in combination with two aldehyde molecules, produces a reddish purple additional complex. The chemical mechanism is not known but it is suggested that with the addition of the aldehydes the reagent undergoes a molecular rearrangement to form an intensely coloured quinoid complex. This final product is not basic fuchsin and varies in colour with the different aldehydes produced by oxidation.

An occasional problem with the preparation of Schiff's reagent is that some batches of basic fuchsin fail to work satisfactorily. The dye should be added to the water at 50°C (see p. 19).

Feulgen's stain for DNA

Another application of Schiff's reagent is in the Feulgen 'nucleal' method for demonstrating deoxyribonucleic acid (DNA). Gentle hydrolysis of DNA leads to the production of aldehyde groups from the deoxyribose component of the DNA molecule; the aldehydes give the characteristic purple colour with Schiff's reagent. Hydrolysis is achieved by treatment of the section by N–HCl at 60°C, and the hydrolysis time needed varies with the fixative used (e.g. Zenker's fixative needs 5 minutes hydrolysis, Susa's fixative 18 minutes). Bouin's fixative is not recommended because of the excessive hydrolysis it causes during fixation. For fuller details of hydrolysis times with various fixatives see Table 2.3. Under- or over-hydrolysis leads to weakening of staining intensity with Schiff's reagent. The method is considered specific for DNA.

Table 2.3. Hydrolysis times with various fixatives

Fixative	Time in minutes	Fixative	Time in minutes
Bouin	Not recommended	Formalin	8
Carnoy	6	Formol sublimate	8
Ethanol	5	Helly	8
		Susa	18
Flemming's	16	Zenker	5

Ribonucleic acid (RNA) is *not* demonstrated by the Feulgen reaction and is usually stained by the methyl green pyronin technique (Unna–Pappenheim). This demonstrates both RNA and DNA (for method see p. 119). Fluorescent staining can also be used to demonstrate DNA and RNA in frozen sections using acridine orange (Bertalanffy and Bickis, 1956).

Extraction techniques allow specific controls to be used for the methods listed in Table 2.4. Two types of extraction are available, enzymatic and

Table 2.4. Methods to demonstrate nucleic acids

Method	Demonstrates	Page
Feulgen	DNA	23
Methyl green pyronin	RNA, DNA	119
Acridine orange	RNA, DNA on frozen sections and smears only	—
Gallocyanin chrome alum	RNA, DNA	—
NAH Feulgen (Pearse, 1951)	DNA	—
Deoxyribonuclease	Extracts DNA only	—
Ribonuclease	Extracts RNA only	—

chemical. The best results are obtained by enzymatic digestion but pure enzymes must be used. Ribonuclease will extract RNA from sections when used at 37°C for one hour; DNA is unaffected. Deoxyribonuclease will extract

Table 2.5. Routine Staining of Mucosubstances

Mucosubstances	Example	Alcian★ blue	Azure A Tol. blue	PAS	Others
Polysaccharides	Glycogen	–	–	+ve	Best's, Bauer–Feulgen
Neutral mucosubstances	Neutral glycoprotein	–	–	+ve	
Acid mucosubstances					
Acidic sulphated					
(a) Connective tissue (synonym: acidic, strongly sulphated).	In heart valves	pH 2.5 weak or –ve / pH 0.5 blue++	pH 2.0 + / pH 6.0 –	?–ve	
(b) Epithelial (synonym: acidic, weakly sulphated).	In colonic goblet cells	pH 2.5 blue / pH 0.5 weak blue	pH 2.0 + / pH 6.0 ±	?–ve	Mucicarmine
Acidic non-sulphated					
(a) Hexuronic acid rich	In synovium, mesothelium etc.	pH 2.5 blue / pH 0.5 –ve	pH 2.0 – / pH 6.0 +	–ve	Mucicarmine
(b) Sialic acid rich	In mucous cells of submandibular salivary glands	pH 2.5 blue++ / pH 0.5 –ve	pH 2.0 – / pH 6.0 +	+ve	Mucicarmine
Mucoproteins and glycoproteins	In basement membranes	–	–	+ve	Protein method
Mucolipids	Cerebrosides	–	–	+ve	Lipid method if frozen section

★ For results with 'critical concentration' technique see page 21.

DNA from sections, also at 37°C, but requires up to 24 hours, while RNA is unaffected.

Table 2.5 summarises the routine staining procedures for mucosubstances.

STAINING METHODS
PAS reaction
SOLUTION
Schiff's reagent (de Tomasi, 1936)

Basic fuchsin	1 g
N Hydrochloric acid	20 ml
Sodium metabisulphite	1 g
Activated charcoal	2 g
Distilled water	200 ml

Boil the distilled water, allow to cool to 80°C, and into this dissolve the basic fuchsin. As the solution cools filter, and at 50°C add the hydrochloric acid. When 25°C is reached add the sodium metabisulphite. Store in dark overnight. Add the activated charcoal, shake for 1 minute and filter; the filtrate should be clear. Store in a dark bottle at 4°C.

METHOD
1. Place sections in xylol, then down to water.
2. Rinse in distilled water.
3. Oxidise in 1 per cent periodic acid for 10 minutes.
4. Wash well in distilled water.
5. Treat with Schiff's reagent for 10 minutes.
6. Wash in running tap water for 10 minutes.
7. Stain nuclei in Mayer's haemalum for 5 minutes.
8. Differentiate in 1 per cent acid alcohol if necessary.
9. Wash well in tap water.
10. Dehydrate through graded alcohols to xylol, mount in DPX.

RESULTS
PAS-positive material: *red*.
Nuclei: *blue*.

NOTES
Discard the solution should it develop a pink coloured tint.

Standard alcian blue for acid mucosubstances
(Steedman, 1950—modified)
As previously discussed alcian blue can be used to demonstrate the various acid mucosubstances. The method given below is the general method which, when used at pH 2.5–3.0, will demonstrate the majority of acid mucosubstances.

SOLUTION
Alcian blue

Alcian blue	1 g
3 per cent acetic acid	100 ml

METHOD
1. Place sections in xylol, then down to water.
2. Stain in alcian blue for 5–10 minutes.
3. Wash in running tap water.
4. Counterstain if required in 1 per cent neutral red or Mayer's carmalum.
5. Wash in tap water.
6. Dehydrate, clear and mount in DPX.

RESULTS
Acid mucosubstances: *blue-green*.
Nuclei: *red*.

NOTES
1. Stain will deteriorate with time.
2. The alcian blue solution should be at pH 2.6.
3. Filter solution before use.

Aldehyde fuchsin alcian blue (Gomori, 1950; Spicer and Meyer, 1960)
  Aldehyde fuchsin is not specific for mucosubstances, but is useful for demonstrating acidic sulphated mucosubstances whilst not reacting with the acidic non-sulphated mucosubstances. For this reason the combined aldehyde fuchsin-alcian blue, as suggested by Spicer and Meyer (1960) and reiterated by Cook (1972), is useful for distinguishing the types of acidic mucosubstances.

SOLUTIONS
Aldehyde fuchsin

Basic fuchsin	1 g
60 per cent alcohol	100 ml
Hydrochloric acid (concentrated)	1 ml
Paraldehyde	2 ml

To the basic fuchsin and alcohol add the hydrochloric acid and paraldehyde. Allow the solution to stand for 2 days by which time the blue colour will have developed.

Alcian blue
  See page 19.

METHOD
1. Place sections in xylol then down to 70 per cent alcohol.
2. Stain in aldehyde fuchsin for 20 minutes.
3. Rinse in 70 per cent alcohol.
4. Wash in running tap water.
5. Stain in alcian blue for 5 minutes.
6. Wash in running tap water.
7. Dehydrate, clear and mount in DPX.

RESULTS
Acidic strongly sulphated mucosubstances: *deep purple*.
Acidic weakly sulphated mucosubstances: *purple*.
Acidic non-sulphated mucosubstances: *blue-green*.

NOTES
   Aldehyde fuchsin is a notoriously capricious solution usually due to the paraldehyde it contains. The stain itself will deteriorate with time. Store at 4°C.

Alcian blue with varying electrolyte concentrations
(Scott and Dorling, 1965)

SOLUTIONS

Alcian blue	50 mg
Acetate buffer pH 5.8	100 ml

For varying the electrolyte concentrations the following amounts of magnesium chloride should be added to each 100 ml of alcian blue (A.B.):
for 0.06M add 1.20 g
for 0.3M add 6.10 g
for 0.5M add 10.15 g
for 0.7M add 14.20 g
for 0.9M add 18.30 g

METHOD
1. Bring sections to water.
2. Stain in the various alcian blue solutions overnight.
3. Wash.
4. Counterstain in neutral red for 3 minutes.
5. Wash.
6. Dehydrate through graded alcohols to xylol.
7. Mount in DPX.

RESULTS
   With the varying electrolyte concentrations the only substances stained are as follows:
A.B. with 0.06M $MgCl_2$: *carboxylated and sulphated mucins*.
A.B. with 0.3M $MgCl_2$: *weakly and strongly sulphated mucins*.
A.B. with 0.5M $MgCl_2$: *strongly sulphated mucins only*.
A.B. with 0.7M $MgCl_2$: *highly sulphated connective tissue mucins*.
A.B. with 0.9M $MgCl_2$: *keratan sulphate only*.

NOTES
1. Sections should be stained for at least 4 hours; overnight staining gives a good result.
2. Some background staining may occur, especially with the low molarity solutions.

Mucicarmine (Southgate, 1927)
   Mucicarmine is a much used, but an empirical and, at times, a capricious

method, that stains the majority of the sulphated mucosubstances, but without contributing to the histochemistry of carbohydrates.

SOLUTION

Carmine	1 g
Aluminium hydroxide	1 g
Aluminium chloride	0.5 g
50 per cent alcohol	100 ml

Dissolve carmine and aluminium hydroxide in the alcohol, mix well by shaking, then add the aluminium chloride. Boil solution for 3 minutes in a *500 ml conical flask*. Allow to cool and make up to 100 ml with the 50 per cent alcohol. Store at 4°C.

METHOD
1. Place sections in xylol, then down to water.
2. Stain nuclei in Mayer's haemalum for 10 minutes.
3. Wash well in running tap water.
4. Differentiate in 1 per cent acid alcohol.
5. Wash well in running tap water.
6. Stain in mucicarmine solution for 20–30 minutes.
7. Wash in running tap water.
8. Dehydrate, clear and mount in DPX.

RESULTS
Mucosubstances: *red*.
Nuclei: *blue*.

NOTES
Use solution as above or diluted 1:4 with distilled water.

Alcian blue PAS (Mowry, 1956)
Acid and neutral mucins.

SOLUTIONS
Alcian blue

Alcian blue	1 g
Acetic acid	3 ml
Distilled water	97 ml

1 per cent periodic acid

Periodic acid	1 g
Distilled water	100 ml

Schiff's reagent
See page 19.

METHOD
1. Place sections in xylol and then down to water.
2. Stain in alcian blue solution for 5 minutes.

3. Wash well in tap water.
4. Treat with 1 per cent periodic acid for 5 minutes.
5. Wash in distilled water.
6. Place in Schiff's reagent for 8 minutes.
7. Wash in running tap water for 10 minutes.
8. Dehydrate through graded alcohols to xylol.
9. Mount in DPX.

RESULTS
Acid mucopolysaccharides: *blue.*
Neutral mucins: *magenta.*
Mixtures of acid and neutral mucins: *purple.*

NOTES
   A nuclear counterstain can be employed, but tends to obscure background staining of alcian blue.

Feulgen nucleal reaction for DNA (Feulgen and Rossenbeck, 1924)

SOLUTIONS
N *Hydrochloric acid*

Hydrochloric acid (concentrated)	8.5 ml
Distilled water	91.5 ml

Schiff's reagent
   See page 19.

METHOD
   1. Place sections in xylol, then down to water.
   2. Rinse sections in N-HCl at room temperature.
   3. Hydrolyse sections in N-HCl at 60°C (see Table 2.3.)
   4. Rinse in N-HCl at room temperature.
   5. Rinse in distilled water.
   6. Transfer sections to Schiff's reagent for 45 minutes.
   7. Drain and transfer to 3 changes of sulphurous acid rinse (see p. 106) for 2 minutes each.
   8. Wash in running tap water 5 minutes.
   9. Counterstain in 1 per cent aqueous light green for 2 minutes.
  10. Wash in tap water.
  11. Dehydrate through graded alcohols to xylene and mount in DPX.

RESULTS
DNA: *magenta.*
Cytoplasm: *green.*

NOTES
1. Preheat the N-HCl to 60°C before use.
2. The correct time for hydrolysis must be used.
3. The counterstain is optional, it may be omitted or a different one used.
4. Specificity can be confirmed by extraction methods.

REFERENCES

BERTALANFFY, L. VON & BICKIS, I. (1956). Identification of cytoplasmic basophilia (ribonucleic acid) by fluorescence microscopy. *J. Histochem. Cytochem.*, **4**, 481.

COOK, H. C. (1972). *Human Tissue Mucins* (Laboratory Aid Series), ed. Baker, F. J. London: Butterworths.

FEULGEN, R. & ROSSENBECK, H. (1924). Mikroskopisch-chemischer Nachweis einer Nucleinsaure vom Typus der Thymonucleinsaure und die darauf beruhende elektive Farbung von Zellkernen in mikroskopischen Praparaten. *Hoppe-Seyler's Z. Physiol. Chem.*, **135**, 203.

GOLDSTEIN, D. J. & HOROBIN, R. W. (1974). Rate factors in staining by alcian blue. *Histochem. J.*, **6**, 157.

GOMORI, G. (1950). Aldehyde fuchsin. A new stain for elastic tissue. *Amer. J. clin. Path.*, **20**, 665.

HOTCHKISS, R. D. (1948). A microchemical reaction resulting in the staining of polysaccharide structures in fixed tissue preparations. *Arch. Biochem.*, **16**, 131.

JACKSON, E. L. & HUDSON, C. S. (1937). Application of the cleavage type of oxidation by periodic acid to starch and cellulose. *J. Amer. chem. Soc.*, **50**, 2049.

LILLIE, R. D. (1947a). Studies on the preservation and the histologic demonstration of glycogen. *Bull. int. Assoc. med. Mus.*, **27**, 23.

LILLIE, R. D. (1947b). Reticulin staining with Schiff reagent after oxidation by acidified sodium periodate. *J. Lab. clin. Med.*, **32**, 910.

McMANUS, J. F. A. (1948). Periodic acid routine applied to kidney. *Amer. J. Path.*, **24**, 643.

MALAPRADE, L. (1934). Etude de l'action des polyalcools sur l'acide periodique et les periodates alcalins. *Bull. Soc. chim. Fr.*, 5 series **1**, 833.

MEYER, K. (1966). Problems of histochemical identification of carbohydrate rich tissue components. *J. Histochem. Cytochem.*, **14**, 605.

MOWRY, R. W. (1956). Alcian blue techniques for the histochemical study of acidic carbohydrates. *J. Histochem. Cytochem.*, **4**, 407.

PEARSE, A. G. E. (1951). A review of modern methods in histochemistry. *J. Clin. Path.*, **4**, 1.

PEARSE, A. G. E. (1968). *Histochemistry, Theoretical and Applied*, 3rd edition Vol. 1. London: Churchill.

SCOTT, J. E. & DORLING, J. (1965). Differential staining of acid glycosaminoglycans (mucopolysaccharides) by alcian blue in salt solutions. *Histochemie*, **5**, 221.

SOUTHGATE, H. W. (1927). Note on preparing mucicarmine. *J. Path. Bact.*, **30**, 729.

SPICER, S. S. (1960). A correlative study of the histochemical properties of rodent acid mucopolysaccharides. *J. Histochem. Cytochem.*, **8**, 18.

SPICER, S. S. & MAYER, D. B. (1960). Histochemical differentiation of acid mucopolysaccharides by the means of combined aldehyde fuschin-alcian blue staining. *Tech. Bull. Reg. med. Technol.*, **30**, 53.

SPICER, S. S., LEPPI, T. J. & STOWARD, P. J. (1965). Suggestions for a histochemical terminology of carbohydrate-rich tissue components. *J. Histochem. Cytochem.*, **13**, 599.

STEEDMAN, H. F. (1950). Alcian blue 8 GS—a new stain for mucin. *Quart. J. micr. Sci.* **91**, 477.

DE TOMASI, J. A. (1936). Improving the technique of the Feulgen stain. *Stain Technol.*, **11**, 137.

FURTHER READING

BANCROFT, J. D. (1975). *An Introduction to Histochemical Techniques*, 2nd edition. London: Butterworths (in Press).

COOK, H. C. (1972). *Human Tissue Mucins* (Laboratory Aids Series), ed. Baker, F. J. London: Butterworths.

PEARSE, A. G. E. (1968). *Histochemistry, Theoretical and Applied*, Volume 1, pp. 294–381. London: Churchill.

CASSELMANN, W. G. B. (1962). *Histochemical Technique*. London: Methuen.

LAKE, B. D. (1970). The histochemical evaluation of glycogen storage diseases. A review of techniques and their limitations. *Histochem. J.* **2**, 441.

CHAPTER 3

Frozen Sections and Lipids

In certain circumstances paraffin, celloidin, or resin-embedded sections are unsuitable for diagnostic purposes, i.e.

(a) when the diagnosis is required very urgently, and the processing and embedding in paraffin or resin would take too long,

(b) when certain important labile tissue components would be either dissolved (e.g. lipids) or destroyed (e.g. enzymes) by the reagents and heat used in processing and embedding techniques,

(c) for immunofluorescence studies.

FROZEN SECTIONS

In these situations frozen sections of the tissue must be prepared. The principle is simple: the tissue is rendered rigid by freezing rather than by embedding in paraffin wax or resin; the tissue water acts as the embedding medium and it is therefore capable of being cut into thin sections. This solves both problems, in that the tissue can be adequately frozen in a matter of seconds or a couple of minutes (depending on which method of freezing is used) and sections can be cut immediately on a modified microtome, and subsequently stained. At no stage is the tissue exposed to any organic solvents or other agents which could dissolve or destroy any lipids, enzymes or antibodies in the tissue. In some cases preliminary fixation of the tissue is neither necessary, nor desirable.

The most common uses of frozen section are:

(a) *in routine surgical histology* where an urgent diagnosis is required, perhaps in the middle of a surgical operation. The most common example of this is in the surgical treatment of lumps in the breast. A part or all of the lump is removed and a frozen section is prepared and stained with H & E (Fig. 3.1). Within 5 minutes the pathologist can tell whether the tumour is malignant, in which case the surgeon proceeds to remove all or part of the breast.

(b) for the demonstration of *lipids* in tissues. Some of the more common clinical applications include the detection of fat embolism in brain, the distinction between thecoma (fat-containing) and fibroma of the ovary, the diagnosis of liposarcoma and the investigation of lipid storage diseases. Sections which are to be stained for lipids are best cut on a freezing microtome and stained (e.g. with oil red O) in a free-floating state. Although the cryostat is more convenient and usually gives better quality sections, we feel that technically superior staining results are obtained by the free-floating technique.

(c) for the histochemical demonstration of *enzyme activity*. So far enzyme histochemistry has been little applied in routine histology, but it is a very important research procedure, and more clinical applications will undoubtedly follow. Enzyme methods are now being extensively used in muscle biopsies (see Chap. 11).

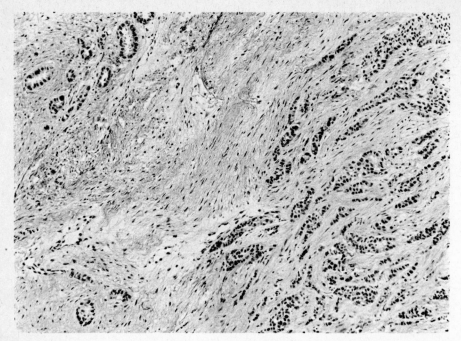

Figure 3.1 Excision biopsy of a lump in the breast; the tissue has been frozen and a section cut in a cryostat. A rapid haematoxylin and eosin stain shows the tumour to be an infiltrating mammary carcinoma with some tubular differentiation. With care and practice, excellent results can be obtained. Magnification (× 252)

(d) for the silver and gold impregnation methods in neurohistology (Cajal, Hortega, etc., see Chap. 6).

(e) for *immunofluorescence studies*. Frozen sections of tissue are essential in the rapidly expanding field of diagnostic immunofluorescence. These are of considerable importance in renal biopsies where the nature and distribution of antibody and antigen–antibody complexes in the glomeruli may have considerable diagnostic significance.

In the future it is likely that a specific method for the histological diagnosis of amyloid will be based upon an immunofluorescent technique.

Freezing techniques

Methods suitable for use with the cryostat are (Bancroft, 1975)
(a) solid carbon dioxide (cardice),
(b) cardice mixtures (cardice, acetone),
(c) carbon dioxide gas,
(d) liquified gases (nitrogen),
(e) cold contact (refrigerated test tubes).
In freezing blocks for the cryostat, consideration should be given to the application of the sections. For histochemical and non-urgent material, the fastest procedure (i.e. liquid nitrogen if available) should always be used. This is certainly the case with muscle biopsies, as artefacts will occur if the rate of freezing is slow. Urgent surgical biopsies are often frozen with cardice or carbon dioxide gas as this does not take the tissue down to extremely low

temperatures (e.g. $-190°C$ with liquid nitrogen) eliminating the need to wait until the tissue warms up to $-20°C$ before cutting.

Tissue that is to be cut on the freezing microtome is frozen with carbon dioxide gas with the conventional freezing microtome or on thermomodules if a thermoelectric attachment is used.

Cutting of frozen sections

FREEZING MICROTOME

This technique has been in use for many years and at one time it was the only way frozen sections were cut in a histology laboratory. The tissue can be either fixed or unfixed. If unfixed tissue is used the knife must be cooled. For convenience, however, the tissue is best fixed. For many years urgent surgical operation specimens were prepared by this technique which commands both skill and experience. Today it is most frequently used for fat stains and work on the central nervous system.

Thermomodule attachment. This is a relatively recent modification of the freezing microtome technique and eliminates the need for freezing by carbon dioxide. A thermomodule is based on the Peltier effect, i.e. that at the junctions of two dissimilar metals heat is absorbed or evolved when a direct current is passed across. These modules are available commercially and are capable of producing temperatures of $-25°C$ on one surface and $+25°C$ on the other. The temperature is controlled by the amount of direct current passed through the module. This gives excellent control of tissue temperature when the block is attached to the cold surface of the module. Once it is known which temperature provides the correct cutting consistency, it can be maintained $\pm 0.1°C$ for as long as required. This has enabled easier cutting, thinner sections and the production of serial sections, which are difficult to obtain with the standard freezing microtome technique. The method is used for fat stains, CNS stains and, where no cryostat is available, for urgent biopsy specimens from the operating theatre.

THE CRYOSTAT

The advent of the cryostat has brought considerable changes to the routine histology laboratory. Urgent biopsy specimens can now be cut more quickly and more conveniently than before, producing thinner sections with less artefact than by any other technique. This is brought about by housing a modified microtome in a refrigerated cabinet, the temperature being maintained at that at which the tissue cuts best (between $-15°C$ and $-20°C$). The cryostat was introduced into the U.K. by Pearse in 1954. Two commercial firms produce the majority of the machines used today in the U.K. Unfixed tissue is frozen outside the cryostat as rapidly as possible using liquid gases or solid carbon dioxide. The microtome is remotely operated and sections are picked up on slides or coverslips. The one drawback to the cryostat is the cutting of fixed material. Two factors cause problems here: at the normal cabinet temperature ($-18°C$ to $-20°C$) cutting of fixed tissue leads to shattering of the sections, and any suitable sections obtained tend to float off the slide during staining. If fixed tissue is to be cut in the cryostat, the tissue should be frozen *slowly* and the temperature of the cabinet *raised* to $-8°C$ to $-10°C$. The slides or coverslips should be coated in a gelatine-formaldehyde solution (see Appendix 2) before being used to pick up the section. The cryostat produces excellent sections for urgent biopsies, histochemistry, CNS tissues and immunofluorescence methods. A suitable method for H & E staining of urgent biopsies is given on p. 31. For further details about the above techniques readers are referred to Clayden (1971) and Bancroft (1975).

LIPIDS

Many of the problems encountered with carbohydrates and mucosubstances (see Chapter 2) are also met with lipids. The recurrent problem is that histochemical techniques are less specific than biochemical methods, and the information derived from both cannot be compared and classified. The nomenclature of lipids is confusing, partly due to a duplication of terms for the same substance. The term lipid as used here includes all natural fats and fat-like materials (Bancroft, 1975). These substances are invariably soluble in organic solvents and a few are soluble in hot water.

Lipids are normal constituents of all tissues either generally in the form of stored lipids (e.g. in adipose tissue) for subsequent energy production, or as specialised lipid structures (e.g. myelin). In many situations they are linked with proteins (lipoproteins) or nitrogenous bases (compound lipids).

In certain diseases excessive amounts of some types of compound lipids accumulate in the cells of the reticulo-endothelial system and sometimes in the neurones of the brain. These disorders are called the 'lipid storage diseases' and are due to the hereditary absence of any of a number of enzymes associated with lipid metabolism. Examples include Niemann–Pick disease (excessive storage of sphingomyelin due to sphingomyelinase deficiency), metachromatic leucodystrophy (excessive galactosyl-3-sulphate ceramide storage due to cerebroside sulphatase deficiency), and Gaucher's disease (excessive glucosyl ceramide storage due to glucosyl ceramide hydrolase deficiency).

Classification of lipids

As was indicated earlier, lipids are rarely found in isolation in human or animal tissues. They are invariably found as mixtures, usually of several compounds. This intermixture of substances is the reason for the failure of techniques such as differential solubility and, to a lesser degree, staining methods in the identification of specific lipids. The following classification is the currently accepted one. It divides lipids into three main groups: simple lipids (e.g. triglycerides), compound lipids (e.g. phospholipids) and derived lipids (e.g. cholesterol).

Simple lipids are esters of fatty acids such as stearic, palmitic and oleic acids with alcohols. They can be conveniently divided into two types.

(a) Neutral fats—composed of molecules of fatty acid combined with one molecule of glycerol (e.g. triglycerides).

(b) Ester waxes—esters of fatty acids and higher alcohols.

Compound lipids have a nitrogenous base with long-chain fatty acids plus a non-lipid compound.

(a) Phospholipids—lecithin, cephalins, plasmals (acetal phosphatides).

(b) Glycolipids—cerebrosides, gangliosides, sphingomyelin.

Derived lipids are obtained by hydrolysis from simple and compound lipids.

(a) Fatty acids (either saturated or unsaturated)—produced from palmitic or stearic acids (saturated) or oleic acid (unsaturated).

(b) Sterols, e.g. cholesterol—produced by the hydrolysis of ester waxes.

HISTOCHEMICAL DEMONSTRATION OF LIPIDS

FIXATION

The majority of lipids are demonstrated in frozen sections. The most suitable fixative is formaldehyde, in the form of formol saline or formol calcium. Since Baker's acid haematein method requires calcium in the fixative it is worth-while to use Baker's formol calcium fixative in all instances.

Unsuitable fixatives. A number of fixatives *cannot* be used in the demonstration of lipids. These include alcohol, and fixatives containing organic solvents. Fixatives containing mercuric chloride are not recommended as these harden the tissue, making the production of sections difficult. Mercuric chloride, however, can be used as a secondary fixative applied to cut sections when necessary.

EXTRACTION

Pure lipids may be extracted by organic solvents and this technique is used in lipid histochemistry to assist in lipid identification. Lipids found in tissue sections, however, are rarely in a pure state and because of this the results obtained with extraction methods should be viewed with caution. Fresh blocks of tissue 2 mm thick are exposed to solvents for a period of 24 hours with three changes of the solvent. After extraction, sections are stained by the various lipid techniques. Keilig (1944) did a considerable amount of work on the solubilities of lipids and her table of results is frequently quoted (Table 3.1) but should be considered in the light of Pearse's (1968) comments.

Table 3.1. Solubility of lipids

Lipid extracted	Solvent
All lipids	Hot chloroform-methanol
Cerebrosides	Hot acetone
Lecithins and cephalins	Hot ether
Glycerides, cholesterol and esters	Cold acetone

A considerable number of methods are at present available to demonstrate the many different types of lipids in tissue sections. The methods given below are the classical methods which are widely known and have been used for many years. A reappraisal of these methods, including an examination of their specificity, has long been overdue. For a description of this work and details of more up to date and specific lipid methods readers are advised to consult Adams and Bayliss (1974).

The neutral and non-acidic lipids will all be stained by the standard Sudan dyes, but differentiation of the various types is not possible. For the isolation of these different lipids the more specialised techniques (see Table 3.2) must be employed.

Sudan dyes

This is a group of dyes that are soluble in liquid or semi-liquid lipids. These dyes, of which Sudan IV, Sudan black B and oil red O are the most popular, have long been used to demonstrate lipids. Oil red O probably produces the most intense coloration for neutral lipids. The Sudan black B technique appears to stain finer droplets of lipid and according to Pearse (1968) is more soluble in phospholipids.

The dyes are suspended in a solvent in which they are only partially soluble, and when the dye solution is applied to lipids (in which the dye is *more* soluble), transfer of the dye into the lipid occurs. The original dye solvent must not be capable of dissolving appreciable amounts of the lipid in the tissue section. Therefore staining occurs with these lipid-soluble dyes because the dye is more soluble in the lipid in the tissue section than it is in the original solvent. A number of solvents have been used but we consider 60 per cent aqueous triethyl phosphate gives the best results. It is obvious from our knowledge of the staining mechanism that only lipids in liquid or semi-liquid form in the tissues will be stained by these Sudan dye methods. Some lipids present in tissues in solid form can be rendered semi-liquid, and therefore stainable, by raising the temperature at which the method is performed to 37°C, 60°C or even higher.

Nile blue sulphate (Lorrain Smith, 1908; Cain, 1947)

This method is used in the further identification of lipids. It demonstrates whether non-acidic or acidic lipids or both are present in a frozen section. Non-acidic lipids stain red, and acidic lipids (e.g. fatty acids, phospholipids) stain blue.

Acid haematein (Baker, 1946)

This is used to demonstrate phospholipids in frozen sections. It is specific when used with Baker's pyridine extraction technique. The techniques are given on pages 33, and 34. Phospholipids stain dark blue, but are negative after pyridine extraction.

Performic acid Schiff (Pearse, 1951)

This technique demonstrates unsaturated lipids. Lipids which give a positive result with this method and with a Sudan dye can be considered to be unsaturated lipids. This can be confirmed by bromination. Unsaturated lipids stain pink to red.

Plasmal reaction (Feulgen and Voit, 1924; Terner and Hayes, 1961)

This technique may be used to demonstrate plasmalogens (acetal phosphatides) by using mercuric chloride to break the acetal linkage, followed by demonstration of the resultant aldehydes by Schiff's reagent. Acetal phosphatides stain pink to red.

Digitonin method (Windaus, 1910)

This technique is used to demonstrate and distinguish between cholesterol and cholesterol esters. Free cholesterol forms a complex with digitonin, producing birefringent crystals.

Perchloric acid naphthoquinone method (PAN) (Adams, 1961)

This technique has replaced the Schultz method for cholesterol and related substances, and is more sensitive than the original Schultz methods. Cholesterol stains dark blue; this coloration lasts for only a few hours.

Osmium tetroxide

This is not used routinely as a means of demonstrating lipids, but is the basis of the Marchi method for demonstrating degenerate myelin (see Chapter 6, p. 67).

A summary of lipid-staining methods is given in Table 3.2.

Table 3.2. Lipid-staining methods

Method	Demonstrates	Page
Oil red O	Liquid and semi-liquid lipids	32
Sudan black B	Liquid and semi-liquid lipids	32
PAN	Cholesterol and related substances	—
PAS	Glycolipids	19
Performic acid Schiff	Unsaturated lipids	—
Plasmal reaction	Acetal phosphatides	—
Baker's acid haematein	Phospholipids	33
Nile blue sulphate	Acidic lipids (phospholipids, fatty acids)	—
	Non-acidic lipids (triglycerides, cholesterol, glycolipid)	—
Digitonin	Free cholesterol	—
Osmium tetroxide	Lipid material	—
Phosphine 3R (fluorescent)	Simple and compound lipids	—

STAINING METHODS

Haematoxylin and eosin staining for urgent cryostat sections

SOLUTION

Scott's tap water

Potassium bicarbonate	2 g
Magnesium sulphate	20 g
Tap water	1000 ml

METHOD

1. Fix cryostat section in AAF (see Appendix 1) for 30 seconds.
2. Dip in tap water.
3. Place sections in Harris' haematoxylin prewarmed to 37°C, 20 seconds.
4. Rinse in tap water.
5. Dip in 1 per cent acid alcohol.
6. Rinse in Scott's tap water.
7. Rinse in tap water.
8. Stain in 1 per cent eosin for 15 seconds.
9. Rinse in tap water.
10. Dehydrate, clear and mount.

RESULTS

See page 7.

NOTES
1. Some workers prefer to miss the fixation stage.
2. Carazzi's haematoxylin may be used in step 3 as no differentiation is required.

Oil red O for lipids (Lillie and Ashburn, 1943, modified)
SOLUTION

Oil red O	1 g
60 per cent triethyl phosphate	100 ml

The solution is heated to 100°C for 5 minutes and stirred constantly. Filter when hot, then again when cool. The solution keeps well but must be filtered before use.

METHOD
1. Place frozen sections in 60 per cent triethyl phosphate.
2. Stain in oil red O solution for 15 minutes.
3. Wash sections in 60 per cent triethyl phosphate for 15–30 seconds.
4. Wash in distilled water.
5. Stain in haematoxylin for 1 minute.
6. Wash in tap water for 5 minutes.
7. Mount in glycerin jelly.

RESULTS

Lipid material: *red.*
Nuclei: *blue.*

NOTES
  This method gives the most intense colour reaction of available Sudan methods.

Sudan black for lipid material (Lison and Dagnelie, 1935, modified)
SOLUTION

Sudan black	1 g
60 per cent triethyl phosphate	100 ml

Heat to 100°C for 5 minutes stirring constantly. The solution is filtered when hot and again when cool. The stain keeps well but must be filtered before use.

METHOD
1. Place sections in 60 per cent triethyl phosphate.
2. Stain in Sudan black solution for 10 minutes.
3. Rinse in 60 per cent triethyl phosphate for 15–30 seconds.
4. Wash in distilled water.
5. Stain nuclei in Mayer's carmalum for 3 minutes.
6. Rinse in tap water.
7. Mount in glycerin jelly.

RESULTS
Lipid material: *black.*
Nuclei: *red.*

Baker's acid haematein for phospholipids (Baker, 1946)

SOLUTIONS
Postchroming solution

Potassium dichromate	5 g
Calcium chloride	1 g
Distilled water	100 ml

Acid haematein

Haematein	50 g
1 per cent sodium iodate	1 ml
Distilled water	48 ml

Heat the solution to boiling point, then cool. When at room temperature add 1 ml acetic acid.

Borax-ferricyanide

Potassium ferricyanide	250 mg
Sodium tetraborate	250 mg
Distilled water	100 ml

METHOD

1. Place blocks of tissue in 10 per cent formol calcium for 6–12 hours at room temperature.
2. Transfer tissue to postchroming solution for 18 hours at room temperature.
3. Transfer to fresh postchroming solution for 24 hours at 60°C.
4. Wash in running tap water overnight.
5. Cut frozen sections at 10μ thick.
6. Postchrome sections for 1 hour at 60°C.
7. Wash well in distilled water.
8. Stain in acid haematein for 5 hours at 37°C.
9. Differentiate in borax ferricyanide solution for 18 hours at 37°C.
10. Wash in tap water for 10 minutes.
11. Mount in glycerin jelly.

RESULTS
Phospholipids: *dark blue*.

NOTE
   The nucleoproteins and cerebrosides may also stain dark blue.

Pyridine extraction (Baker, 1946)

SOLUTION
Dilute Bouin's fixative

Picric acid (aqueous saturated)	50 ml
Formaldehyde	10 ml
Glacial acetic acid (concentrated)	5 ml
Distilled water	35 ml

METHOD
1. Fix block of tissue in dilute Bouin's fixative for 20 hours.
2. Wash in 70 per cent alcohol for 1 hour.
3. Wash in 50 per cent alcohol for 30 minutes.
4. Wash in running tap water for 30 minutes.
5. Transfer tissue to pyridine at 20°C for 1 hour.
6. Transfer to fresh pyridine at 20°C for 1 hour.
7. Transfer to fresh pyridine at 60°C for 24 hours.
8. Wash in running tap water for 2 hours.
9. Transfer to step 2 of Baker's haematein method.

RESULTS
After the above treatment phospholipids will be removed.

REFERENCES

ADAMS, C. W. M. (1961). A perchloric acid–napthoquinone method for the histochemical location of cholesterol. *Nature*, **192**, 331.

ADAMS, C. W. M. & BAYLISS, O. B. (1974). Lipid histochemistry. In *Techniques of Biochemical and Biophysical Morphology*, ed. Glick, D. & Rosenbaum, R., Vol. II, Ch. New York: Wiley.

BANCROFT, J. D. (1975). *An Introduction to Histochemical Technique*, 2nd edition. London: Butterworths (in Press).

BAKER, J. R. (1946). The histochemical recognition of lipine. *Quart. J. micr. Sci.*, **87**, 441.

CAIN, A. J. (1947). The use of nile blue in the examination of lipids. *Quart. J. micr. Sci.*, **88**, 467.

CLAYDEN, E. C. (1971). Practical Section Cutting and Staining, 5th edition. Edinburgh & London: Churchill Livingstone.

FEULGEN, R. & VOIT, K. (1924). Uber einen weitverbreiteten festen aldehyd. *Pflsluger's Arch. Ges., Physiol.*, **206**, 389.

KEILIG, I. (1944). Uber spezifitatsbreite und grundlagen der markscheidenfarbungen nach untersuchungen an fraktioniert extralierten gehirnen. *Virchows Arch. path. Anat.*, **312**, 405.

LILLIE, R. D. & ASHBURN, L. L. (1943). Super-saturated solutions of fat stains in dilute isopropanyl for demonstration of acute fatty degenerations not shown by Herxheimer technique. *Arch. Path.*, **36**, 432.

LISON, L. & DAGNELIE, J. (1935). Methodes nouvelles de colouration de la Myeline. *Bull. Histol. Techn. Micr.*, **12**, 85.

LORRIAIN SMITH, J. (1908). On the simultaneous staining of neutral fat and fatty acid by oxazine dyes. *J. Path. Bact.*, **12**, 1.

PEARSE, A. G. E. (1951). A review of modern methods in histochemistry. *J. clin. Path.*, **4**, 1.

PEARSE, A. G. E. (1968). *Histochemistry, Theoretical and Applied*, Vol. 1, pp. 13–27, 398–447. London: Churchill.

TERNER, G. Y. & HAYES, E. R. (1961). Histochemistry of plasmalogens. *Stain Technol.*, **36**, 265.

WINDAUS, T. (1910). Ueber die quantitative bestimmung des cholesterins und der cholesterinester in einigen normulen und pathologischen nieren. *Z. phys. Chem.*, **65**, 110.

FURTHER READING

ADAMS, C. W. M. (1965). *Neurohistochemistry*. London: Elsevier.

CHAPTER 4
Connective Tissues

Collagen fibres

Collagen is a fibrous protein produced by fibroblasts. It is eosinophilic, and when it is recently formed or present in small quantities, its fibrillary nature is usually obvious; when old, and present as large masses, it may appear more homogeneous. It is usually easily recognisable on an H & E stained section; however, in certain circumstances it may be necessary to apply other staining techniques to confirm that a particular mass of tissue is fibroblastic rather than, say, composed of smooth muscle cells. An intimate relationship between the individual cells and demonstrable collagen fibres confirms the fibroblastic nature of the tissue. Stains particularly suitable for this purpose are (a) the van Gieson stain (which stains collagen pinkish-red and muscle fibres yellow) and (b) Masson's trichrome method (which stains collagen green and muscle fibres red); for almost all purposes we prefer the van Gieson stain. An example of a situation in which these stains may be useful is when attempting to decide whether a spindle-celled tumour is a fibrosarcoma or a leiomyosarcoma.

Collagen is birefringent and can be seen under a polarising microscope in either stained or unstained sections. It is a difficult component of tissue to cut, and tissue blocks containing much collagen require careful processing.

Muscle

Muscle cell cytoplasm of all types stains yellow by the van Gieson stain and red by Masson's trichrome. The special stains and histochemical methods useful in the diagnosis of certain diseases of striated muscle by muscle biopsy are dealt with in some detail in Chapter 11.

Two other topics are worth mentioning under this heading, namely the demonstration of cross-striations in tumour cells, and attempts to demonstrate the earliest changes of muscle cell necrosis in very early myocardial infarction.

It is widely held that such rare tumours as rhabdomyosarcoma and the rhabdomyoblast-containing mixed mesodermal tumours can only be diagnosed with certainty if undoubted cross-striations can be demonstrated in some of the tumour cells, and that special stains are usually necessary to demonstrate these cross-striations. In our opinion neither of these beliefs is necessarily valid: the malignant striated muscle cell has many other characteristic features which, taken with a compatible clinical story (and a little common sense), are enough to make a diagnosis. The regular striations are probably the first feature to disappear as a neoplastic striated muscle cell becomes less well differentiated. Nevertheless, cross-striations must be carefully sought in such tumours, the tumour cells around small blood vessels being the most fruitful areas to search. Special stains are usually unnecessary, a well-stained H & E is all that is required. The best stain for the demonstration of cross-striations, however, is *Heidenhain's iron haematoxylin* (see Fig. 1.1, p. 3); unfortunately this method involves tiresome and careful differentiation of the suspected muscle cells under microscopic control. As such, of course, it is virtually useless as a 'search' stain but is rewarding and aesthetically pleasing when one wishes to produce clear photographs of cross-striations in a proven case. The PTAH method has some value as a 'search' stain, since any cross-striations present are slightly emphasised and may be more quickly and easily spotted than on an H & E stain. The method owes its value to the fact that accurate differentiation under microscopic control is not necessary.

The early histological diagnosis of myocardial infarction at necropsy has always been a problem, since the earliest changes detectable with ease on an H & E stained section are not visible until about 12 hours after the initiation of the infarct. Earlier changes can be detected in fresh slices of myocardium at necropsy, and in fresh frozen sections, using enzyme histochemical methods. These techniques are based on the fact that one of the earliest changes occurring in infarcted muscle fibres is the loss of intracytoplasmic enzymes; the enzyme method most frequently used is one of the dehydrogenase methods using a tetrazolium salt to produce a formazan reaction product at sites of enzyme activity. Thus normal myocardium shows activity, infarcted myocardium shows no reaction. Areas of myocardial infarction can be detected about 4–6 hours after the infarctive episode. The method is a laborious chore for a non-histochemically oriented laboratory and the necropsy must be performed within a very short time of death for the method to have any hope of success. Although an interesting exercise the methods are of no real value in everyday routine necropsy practice.

Another attempt has been based on the increased fuchsinophilia of recently necrotic muscle fibres. Reports have appeared of the use of such a stain (Berry, 1967), but in our hands results have often proved difficult to interpret, and the conclusions unreliable.

Reticulin

The reticulin framework of a tissue, made up of variably arranged fine interrelated fibres, is invisible in H & E stained sections but may be roughly deduced from the arrangement of the cells. The reticulin pattern can be directly visualised by the use of methods based on silver impregnation. The appearance of the reticulin pattern is particularly useful in the following situations:

(a) *Liver biopsies*, to emphasise cirrhotic changes (Fig. 11.1, p. 123), particularly in borderline cases. Condensation of the reticulin fibres within a lobule betokens liver cell atrophy or necrosis, as in viral hepatitis.

(b) *Lymphoreticular neoplasms*. Complete loss of the normal reticulin pattern is a characteristic feature of diffuse neoplastic infiltration of a lymph node, either by a lymphoreticular neoplasm or by metastatic tumour. Metastatic carcinomas in lymph nodes create their own reticulin network, often in a characteristic pattern. This feature can sometimes be used in the occasional difficult case when it is difficult to distinguish between reticulum cell sarcoma and metastatic anaplastic carcinoma: carcinoma has a recognisable reticulin pattern whilst reticulum cell sarcoma has a fine network, with individual fibres associated with each neoplastic reticulum cell, and not arranged in any repetitive pattern.

(c) *Other tumours*. A reticulin stain may be invaluable in certain tumours, particularly in the *chemodectomas* where a reticulin stain reveals the

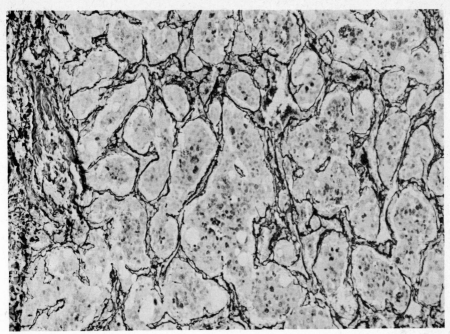

Figure 4.1 A reticulin stain (Gordon and Sweet, with neutral red counterstain) of a tumour removed from the neck of a middle-aged woman. It shows the characteristic reticulin pattern of a chemodectoma ('carotid body tumour'). Magnification (× 392)

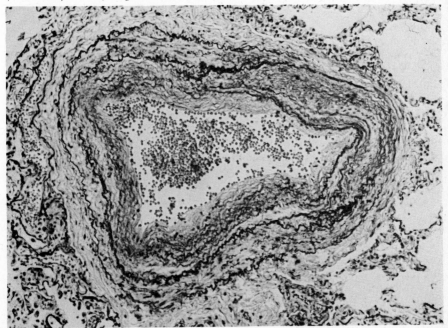

Figure 4.2 An intrapulmonary artery branch from a patient with severe pulmonary hypertension, stained by Weigert's Elastic van Gieson method for elastic fibres. Note the reduplication of the internal elastic lamina and the fibro-elastic intimal thickening. Magnification (× 157)

characteristic arrangement of tumour cells in round clumps ('zellerballen') which is not always apparent on H & E stained sections (Fig. 4.1). Other uses are in angiomas, angiosarcomas and particularly *haemangiopericytomas* where the vascular nature of the tumours, and the relationships of the neoplastic cells to the vessels are easily discernible.

There are many reticulin methods available, of which Gordon and Sweet's, Foot's, and Gomori's are the most popular; we prefer the Gordon and Sweet method.

Many pathologists use no counterstain with reticulin methods; we prefer a light neutral red counterstain.

Elastic fibres

Elastic fibres are strongly eosinophilic, and when they are arranged compactly and in a regular parallel fashion (as in arterial elastic laminae and in the wall of the aorta) they show a refractility which enables them to be fairly easily identified. The particular use of elastic stains is in the study of vascular disease, where such abnormalities of the elastic laminae as splitting and reduplication (hypertensive vascular disease) and breaks (active or old arteritis) are easily detected (Fig. 4.2). They find wide application in renal biopsies where they are invaluable in the diagnosis of such conditions as benign and malignant nephrosclerosis, old episodes of vascular transplant rejection, renal polyarteritis and many other diseases. They are also valuable in the examination of surgically resected abnormal heart valves, where the thin elastic line of the normal valve is still easily distinguished, and the damage caused to it by fibrosis, calcification or infection can be readily assessed.

In almost all its applications to the staining of vessels the elastic stain is best combined with the van Gieson stain, since this method stains the muscle of the arterial media yellow, and any collagen in the abnormal intima stains pink. The peculiar elastotic change in collagen, seen in such conditions as the senile (or solar) elastosis of dermal collagen and in fibrosed heart valves, is also stained by the elastic method.

There are numerous methods available for the demonstration of elastic fibres, many of which are based on resorcin dye complexes. *Weigert's* resorcin–fuchsin method gives excellent results, especially if a long (overnight) incubation in stain is used. Unfortunately the preparation of the stain is tricky and time-consuming and occasionally a complete batch of stain will fail to work for no apparent reason; recent modifications of the method, such as that by Humberstone and Humberstone (1969) have eliminated some of these problems. Verhoeff's elastic stain is the easiest to prepare, quickest to perform, and the most consistent, although it often does not stain the very finest fibres. These are the best elastic methods. Gomori's aldehyde fuchsin stain has been used to demonstrate elastic fibres (it stains fibres deep purple) but because the stain is difficult to prepare, and deteriorates rapidly with time, the method has fallen out of favour.

Basement membranes

Basement membranes are best demonstrated by the PAS and Jones methenamine silver methods. The relative merits of these methods are discussed in the chapter on renal biopsy; the most important application of basement membrane stains is in renal biopsy interpretation.

Fibrin and 'fibrinoid'

Fibrin is an insoluble protein with a long thin molecule; it is a polymer of the soluble protein molecule, fibrinogen, which is a normal component of plasma protein. When fibrinogen leaks out from the vessel lumen into the vessel wall or extravascular space, polymerisation occurs and the insoluble polymer is deposited as fine threads of fibrin. Eventually a complex network of threads may form a large mesh of coarser fibres, occasionally condensing with age into an almost amorphous mass. Old fibrin such as this may occasionally show some of the staining reactions of collagen.

Fibrin is produced in many situations, the commonest being in the exudate resulting from the acute inflammatory reaction, and within blood vessels and heart chambers when thrombus is formed. When vessel walls are acutely damaged, fibrin-like material called 'fibrinoid' replaces part of the wall; this phenomenon is called fibrinoid necrosis and is an important diagnostic feature of many serious diseases.

A discussion of the exact nature of the substance known as 'fibrinoid' is beyond the scope of this book; suffice it to say that it shows all the staining reactions of true fibrin, and is almost certainly derived from plasma proteins.

Fibrin and fibrinoid are stained blue by the PTAH method and bright red by Lendrum's Martius–scarlet–blue (MSB) method, although old fibrin may stain blue; the latter is the stain of choice for fibrin and fibrinoid, and was devised by Lendrum and his colleagues as a means of staining fibrin of all ages. Its application to renal biopsy specimens provided an unexpected bonus in that the blue component of the trichrome stain is a very useful glomerular basement membrane and mesangium stain. Concentrated protein solutions, such as may be seen in renal tubules as casts, are also stained red by the MSB method. Like many of the trichrome methods it can be a little difficult in the hands of the novice, as it is vital to get the correct balance between the various colours. Once the technologist has seen a well-performed MSB and knows what to strive for, the method is simplicity itself and gives consistently good results.

Adipose tissue and intracellular lipids

Lipids are dissolved out of tissues during the passage through the alcohols and organic solvents necessary for the production of a paraffin-embedded section. Frozen sections are therefore necessary to demonstrate intracellular lipid. The special stains used are described in the chapter on frozen sections and lipids (Chap. 3).

Bone and cartilage

Useful special stains to demonstrate particular facets of bone and cartilage structure are described in Chapter 7.

The colour reactions of connective tissue are summarised in Table 4.1.

DEMONSTRATION OF CONNECTIVE TISSUES
Connective tissue stains

The importance of being able to differentiate between the different connective tissue fibres has already been stressed. To demonstrate the many

D

Table 4.1. Connective tissue staining reactions

Connective tissue	Van Gieson	Masson's trichrome	PTAH	MSB	PAS	Reticulin silver method
Osteoid	Red	Variable	Brownish red	Blue	Woven bone—pink	Brown
Cartilage	Unstained/pink	Variable	Brownish red		Pink	
Collagen	Red	Green/blue	Brownish red	Blue	Pink	Grey
Elastic fibres		Pale red	Brownish red	Blue	Weak reaction	Sometimes black
Fibrin	Pale yellow	Red	Blue	Red	Can be pale pink	
Reticulin		Green/blue	Brownish red	Blue	Very weak reaction	Black
Muscle	Yellow	Red	Blue	Red	Weak reaction	Black sarcolemma

components involved in connective tissues, a large number of methods have been evolved. The majority of these methods utilise a number of dyes, either as a combined solution or in sequence. Some connective tissue components are selectively stained but others need pre-treatment to render them suitable for the technique.

Fixation is very important for the majority of trichrome-type methods. The choice of the correct fixative will render the tissue able to retain the dyes. The use of secondary fixation is applied to certain trichrome methods, especially if the original fixative is not the one of choice.

A considerable amount of skill is required in employing trichrome methods since the majority involve a number of stages of differentiation to obtain the correct colour balance. The choice of which method to use is a personal one; the methods which are described here are a few of the many available, but have been totally successful in our hands over the years.

STAINING METHODS

Van Gieson method (van Gieson, 1889)

This long-established method is by far the easiest of the methods to differentiate collagen and muscle. The stain is a mixture of picric acid which stains muscle yellow, and acid fuchsin which stains collagen red-pink.

SOLUTIONS
Van Gieson's stain

1 per cent acid fuchsin	10 ml
Saturated solution of picric acid	90 ml

Dilute with an equal volume of distilled water and boil for 3 minutes to 'ripen'.

METHOD
1. Place sections in xylol, then down to water.
2. Stain in celestine blue for 5 minutes.
3. Rinse in water.
4. Stain in Mayer's haemalum for 5 minutes.
5. Wash in water to blue, 5 minutes.
6. Stain in van Gieson solution for 3 minutes.
7. Rinse rapidly in distilled water, and blot.
8. Dehydrate rapidly through graded alcohols to xylol.
9. Mount in DPX.

RESULTS
Collagen: *red-pink.*
Muscle: *yellow.*
Nuclei: *blue-black.*

NOTES
1. The red component is removed by water; if the tap water is alkaline it will remove the red stain very rapidly; in this case distilled water should be used if it is considered necessary.
2. The yellow stain is removed by alcohols.
3. Van Gieson stain will remove the haematoxylin if left on for too long.

Reticulin method (Gordon and Sweet, 1936)
   This reticulin method is probably the most reliable of the many methods available; sections rarely become detached from the slide, a problem with some other reticulin methods. It is a simple silver-reduction method.

SOLUTIONS
Acid permanganate

0.5 per cent aqueous potassium permanganate	50 ml
3 per cent sulphuric acid	2.5 ml

Silver solution

10 per cent silver nitrate	5 ml
3 per cent sodium hydroxide	5 ml
Ammonia	
Glass–distilled water	50 ml

To the silver nitrate add ammonia drop by drop until the precipitate is not quite dissolved, then add the sodium hydroxide. Redissolve the precipitate which forms by adding ammonia drop by drop until only a faint opalescence remains. Make the volume up to 50 ml with glass–distilled water, filter into a dark bottle.

METHOD

1. Place sections in xylol, then down to water.
2. Oxidise sections in acid permanganate solution for 5 minutes.
3. Wash in water.
4. Place in 1 per cent oxalic acid to bleach section.
5. Wash in tap water, followed by distilled water.
6. Mordant in 2 per cent iron alum for 15 minutes.
7. Wash in 2 or 3 changes of distilled water.
8. Impregnate in silver solution for 5 seconds.
9. Wash in 2 changes of distilled water.
10. Reduce in 10 per cent aqueous neutral formalin for 30 seconds.
11. Wash in distilled water, followed by tap water.
12. Tone in 0.2 per cent gold chloride.
13. Wash in tap water.
14. Fix in 5 per cent sodium thiosulphate for 5 minutes.
15. Wash well in tap water.
16. Dehydrate, clear and mount.

RESULTS

Reticulin fibres: *black*.
Collagen: *grey*.

NOTES

1. All silver solutions should be made up in chemically clean glassware.
2. The time in the silver solution varies with the age of the solution. If staining is too dense repeat method from step 6.
3. Toning may be omitted.
4. A counterstain may be employed if required between steps 15 and 16 using 1 per cent neutral red.

Trichrome stain (Masson, 1929, modified)

This technique was a development of the original Mallory stain. In turn many modifications of Masson's method exist. Fixation plays an important role with this technique; the method will work after any fixative but superior results are obtained with formol sublimate, Zenker's or Bouin's fixatives (see Appendix 1). If formol saline is the primary fixative then secondary fixation should be employed. Formalin-fixed sections mordanted for an hour or longer in saturated alcoholic picric acid containing 3 per cent mercuric chloride will give enhanced staining.

SOLUTIONS

Ponceau fuchsin	Ponceau 2R	0.7 g
	Acid fuchsin	0.35 g
	Glacial acetic acid	1.0 ml
	Distilled water	99 ml
Acid water	Glacial acetic acid	0.5 ml
	Distilled water	99.5 ml
Light green	Light green	2.0 g
	Glacial acetic acid	2.0 ml
	Distilled water	98.0 ml

METHOD
1. Place sections in xylol, then down to water.
2. Stain sections in Weigert's iron haematoxylin for 20 minutes (see p. 6) or use the celestine blue–haemalum routine.
3. Wash in tap water.
4. Differentiate in 1 per cent acid alcohol.
5. Wash in tap water.
6. Stain in Ponceau fuchsin solution for 5 minutes.
7. Rinse in acid water solution.
8. Differentiate in 1 per cent phosphomolybdic acid till collagen is pale pink and muscle and fibrin are still bright red, approximately 5 minutes.
9. Rinse in acid water solution.
10. Stain in light green solution till collagen is green, 2–5 minutes.
11. Wash well in acid water.
12. Dehydrate, clear and mount.

RESULTS
Collagen: *green.*
Muscle: *red.*
Fibrin: *red.*
RBC: *red.*
Nuclei: *blue–black.*

NOTES
1. The method requires considerable skill for the most successful result. The choice of fixative will lengthen or shorten staining times but these should always be controlled microscopically in any case.
2. Acid water is used to prevent the dye washing out.
3. Aniline blue can be substituted for light green if required.

Weigert's elastic stain (Weigert, 1898, modified; Moore, 1943)
Many variants exist of the original 1898 method. A number of these employ staining times of up to 4 hours, and in some other methods overnight staining is preferred. The methods using overnight staining utilise more stable solutions and appear to stain very fine fibres.

SOLUTIONS

Elastic stock solution

Crystal violet	2.5 g
Basic fuchsin	2.5 g
Dextrin	1.0 g
Resorcin	10.0 g
Distilled water	500 ml
30 per cent aqueous ferric chloride (anhydrous)	62.0 ml
Distilled water (for washing)	8–10 l
Absolute ethyl alcohol	550 ml
Concentrated hydrochloric acid	20 ml

Heat the distilled water to *nearly* boiling in a large evaporating basin. Mix the dyes and dextrin and dissolve in the hot water. Add the resorcin and bring to the boil. When boiling add slowly the *freshly* prepared ferric chloride solution, stirring continuously with a glass rod. It is important to keep the mixture boiling, though not too vigorously. Continue boiling and stirring for a further 2 minutes or so to coarsen the precipitate. Cool and filter through a Buchner funnel and filter flask attached to the suction pump. Wash the deposit with distilled water until the drips are colourless and the bulk of the filtrate a clear azure blue. Usually 8–10 litres is sufficient. The filter paper is now removed and dried overnight in the incubator, when the deposit is scraped off and dissolved in 550 ml of absolute ethyl alcohol (to which has been added 1 ml of concentrated hydrochloric acid), by simmering on an electric hot plate or water bath for 30 minutes or so. Cool and filter, then add 19 ml concentrated hydrochloric acid and allow to stand 24–48 hours before use, when the colour should be a dark greenish-blue.

Staining solution

Stock solution	35 ml
70 per cent alcohol	30 ml

These amounts may have to be varied slightly with each fresh batch of stain.

Acid permanganate   See page 41.

Van Gieson   See page 40.

METHOD
1. Place sections in xylol, then down to water.
2. Treat sections with acid permanganate for 5 minutes.
3. Wash in tap water.
4. Bleach in 1 per cent oxalic acid till clear.
5. Wash in tap water.
6. Rinse in 95 per cent alcohol.
7. Stain in elastic stain overnight.
8. Rinse in 95 per cent alcohol.
9. Differentiate in acid alcohol until only elastic fibres are stained.
10. Wash well in tap water.
11. Stain sections in celestine blue for 5 minutes.
12. Rinse in tap water.
13. Stain sections in Mayer's haemalum for 5 minutes.
14. Wash well in tap water.
15. Stain in van Gieson for 3 minutes.
16. Very rapidly rinse in distilled water and blot.
17. Dehydrate, clear and mount in DPX.

RESULTS
Elastic fibres: *blue-black*.
Collagen: *red*.
Muscle: *yellow*.
Nuclei: *blue-black*.

Martius–scarlet–blue method (MSB) (Lendrum et al, 1962)

This is an outstanding method for the demonstration of fibrin; to obtain the best results from this method the tissue must be fixed in formal sublimate for a period in excess of one week. If this is not possible then secondary fixation with formal sublimate should be employed. For sections fixed in other agents, treatment with 3 per cent mercuric chloride in saturated alcoholic picric acid will greatly enhance the staining.

SOLUTIONS

Martius yellow

Martius yellow	0.5 g
Phosphotungstic acid	2.0 g
95 per cent alcohol	100 ml

Brilliant crystal scarlet 6R

Brilliant crystal scarlet 6R	1.0 g
Distilled water	97.5 ml
Glacial acetic acid	2.5 ml

Soluble blue

Soluble blue	0.5 g
Distilled water	99 ml
Acetic acid	1 ml

METHOD
1. Place sections in xylol, then down to water.
2. Remove mercury pigment.
3. Stain nuclei in celestine blue for 5 minutes.
4. Briefly wash in tap water.
5. Stain in Mayer's haemalum for 5 minutes.
6. Lightly differentiate in acid alcohol.
7. Wash well in tap water.
8. Rinse in 95 per cent alcohol.
9. Stain in Martius yellow solution for 2 minutes.
10. Rinse in distilled water.
11. Stain in brilliant crystal scarlet 6R solution for 10 minutes.
12. Rinse in distilled water.
13. Treat with 1 per cent phosphotungstic acid (this will differentiate the red stain) for 3–5 minutes.
14. Rinse in distilled water.
15. Stain in soluble blue solution for 5–10 minutes.
16. Rinse in 1 per cent acetic acid.
17. Blot dry, dehydrate in absolute alcohol, clear in xylol and mount in DPX.

RESULTS
Muscle: *red.*
Fibrin: *red.*
Very old fibrin: *purple black.*
Nuclei: *black.*
Erythrocytes: *yellow.*
Other connective tissue including basement membranes: *blue.*

NOTES
1. Thin 3–4 μ sections give the best results.
2. A little practice is needed with this method, after which it is very easy to perform.

Verhoeff's elastic tissue stain (Verhoeff, 1908)
This technique is recommended where there is some urgency in the demonstration of elastic fibres. The method does not stain the fine elastic fibres as well as the Weigert's stain.

SOLUTIONS
Verhoeff's elastic stain

5 per cent unripened alcoholic haematoxylin	30 ml
10 per cent aqueous ferric chloride	12 ml
Lugol's iodine	12 ml

Mix in above order, shaking between each addition.

Van Gieson   See page 40.

METHOD
1. Place sections in xylol, then down to water.
2. Stain in Verhoeff's solution for 15–30 minutes till section is black.
3. Rinse in tap water.
4. Differentiate in 2 per cent ferric chloride until stain is removed from the collagen and muscle but leaving the elastic fibres black.
5. Wash well in tap water.
6. Treat sections in 95 per cent alcohol (to remove non-specific background staining).
7. Rinse in tap water.
8. Counterstain with van Gieson for 1 minute.
9. Rinse very rapidly in distilled water and blot.
10. Dehydrate, clear and mount.

RESULTS
Elastic fibres: *black.*
Nuclei: *grey-black.*
Collagen: *red.*
Muscle: *yellow.*

NOTES
1. The staining solution should be freshly prepared.
2. Prolonged staining with van Gieson will remove the elastic stain.
3. The nuclei are also stained by elastic stain.
4. The differentiation should always be carried out with the aid of a micro-scope. If over-differentiation occurs, the section may be returned to the elastic stain (step 2) and the method repeated.

Table 4.2. Connective tissue staining methods

Method	Demonstrates	Page
Periodic acid Schiff	Basement membranes	19
Methenamine silver	Basement membranes	118
Weigert's elastic stain	Elastic fibres	43
Verhoeff's elastic stain	Elastic fibres	46
Reticulin (Gordon and Sweet's method)	Reticulin fibres	41
Van Gieson	Collagen, muscle	40
Phosphotungstic acid haematoxylin	Collagen, muscle, fibrin	8
Masson's trichrome	Muscle, fibrin, collagen	42
Martius scarlet blue	Fibrin	45
Alcian blue	Acid mucosubstances	19
Oil red O	Lipids	32

REFERENCES

BERRY, C. L. (1967). Myocardial ischaemia in infancy and childhood. *J. clin. Path.*, **20**, 38.

GORDON, H. & SWEET, H. H. (1936). A simple method for the silver impregnation of reticulin. *Amer. J. Path.*, **12**, 545.

HUMBERSTONE, G. C. W. & HUMBERSTONE, F. D. (1969). An elastic tissue stain. *J. med. Lab. Technol.*, **26**, 99.

LENDRUM, A. C., FRASER, D. S., SLIDDERS, W. & HENDERSON, R. (1962). Studies on the character and staining of fibrin. *J. clin. Path.*, **15**, 401.

MASSON, P. (1929). Some histological methods. Trichrome stainings and their preliminary technique. *Bull. int. Ass. med. Mus.*, **12**, 75.

MOORE, G. W. (1943). An improved elastic stain. *Bull. Inst. med. Lab. Technol.* **9**, 9.

van GIESON, I. (1889). Laboratory notes of technical methods for the nervous system. *N.Y. J. Med.*, **50**, 57.

VERHOEFF, F. H. (1908). Some new staining methods of wide applicability. Including a rapid differential stain for elastic tissue. *J. Amer. med. Ass.*, **50**, 876.

WEIGERT, C. (1898). Ueber eine methode zur farbung elastischer fasern. *Zbl. allg. Path. Anat.* **9**, 289.

FURTHER READING

DRURY, R. A. B. & WALLINGTON, E. A. (1967). *Carleton's Histological Technique*, 4th edition. Oxford University Press.

CHAPTER 5
Amyloid

Amyloid is an acellular homogenous eosinophilic material whose exact nature was, until recently, largely a mystery. It acquired its name because it was originally believed to be chemically related to starch.

Distribution of amyloid

The organs most commonly affected by amyloid infiltration are the liver, spleen, kidney and adrenals, but amyloid is frequently present in other organs, both interstitially and in the walls of the vessels of the organ. Hence it can be found in the heart, nerves, bowel wall, skin, alveolar walls and many other sites.

Classification of amyloid

There has been considerable confusion over the classification and nomenclature of the various types of amyloid over the years. The traditional view has been to subdivide amyloid into two main groups, *primary amyloid* and *secondary amyloid*. In the former the amyloidosis is an isolated lesion and is not associated with any disease process; in secondary amyloid there is an associated underlying disease process. Secondary amyloid was much the most common and was frequently associated with chronic inflammatory disease such as tuberculosis, chronic osteomyelitis and empyema. It was widely believed that these two types of amyloid differed in certain important respects, particularly in distribution and staining properties, and the implication was that there was a difference in the structures of the two types of amyloid. Although there was an element of truth in the observations about differences in distribution and staining reactions in some cases, subsequent research on the ultrastructural, physical and chemical characteristics of amyloid has so far demonstrated no difference between primary and secondary types.

Furthermore, amyloid showing the distribution and the weaker staining reactions once held to be associated with the primary type of amyloidosis is often found in association with myelomatosis, and therefore by definition cannot be regarded as primary amyloid.

The problem was further complicated by Missmahl who, using the polarising microscope, believed that amyloid was initially deposited on either reticulin fibres or collagen fibres, and could therefore be classified into *perireticular* and *pericollagenous* types. For many reasons this classification is unworkable (see Cohen, 1967).

CLINICAL ASSOCIATIONS

Amyloid is now probably best considered according to its clinical associations.

(a) *Chronic inflammatory disease*, both infective and non-infective. In the years before antibiotics, chronic suppurative disease such as chronic osteo-myelitis, empyema and bronchiectasis, together with tuberculosis, accounted for most of the cases of amyloidosis in Britain. Now rheumatoid arthritis is probably the most important chronic inflammatory disease leading to the development of amyloidosis.

(b) *Neoplastic disease*. The association between myeloma and the eventual development of amyloidosis is well known. Amyloid material is a constant feature in the stroma of the fascinating tumour, medullary carcinoma of the thyroid. Amyloidosis has also been described as complicating certain other neoplasms, particularly Hodgkin's disease and renal carcinoma.

(c) *Heredo-familial disorders*. Amyloidosis eventually develops in many patients with familial Mediterranean fever, the renal involvement being ultimately fatal. There are numerous examples in the literature of the familial incidence of amyloid, sometimes confined to one organ such as the heart. Other examples are the exotic-sounding familial disorders, Muckle's nephro-pathy and Portuguese neuropathy.

(d) *Senility*. It has long been known that amyloid material is found in the hearts of elderly people ('senile cardiac amyloid'), the incidence rising with increasing age. It is usually found only in microscopic amounts, but occasionally may be in such quantities as to lead to heart failure. Amyloid has also been described in the brains of elderly people with senile dementia, and, a fascinating observation, in the brains of young and middle-aged patients with Alzheimer's disease (a form of pre-senile dementia).

There remains a group of patients with amyloidosis who do not fit into any of the above categories, and in whom there seems to be no associated disease. These are lumped together into the unsatisfactory category of 'primary amyloid', although intensive investigation in some of these cases reveals an occult myeloma.

The nature of amyloid

Ultrastructural studies have shown that amyloid is composed of protein fibrils having constant physical characteristics. Each fibril is about 7.5 nm (75 Å) wide and consists of two electron-dense linear components 2.5 nm (25 Å) wide with a central separation of 2.5 nm (25 Å). The fibrils are usually haphazardly arranged but may occasionally be aggregated into clumps 2–8 fibrils across in which the fibrils are orientated in a parallel fashion (see Fig. 5.2).

An electron-dense beaded rod 10 nm (100 Å) in diameter and up to 400 nm (4000 Å) in length ('P' component) has also been described in amyloid extracts; the rod is divided into transverse bands with a central distance of 4 nm (40 Å). These have not been seen in whole amyloid tissue, and have recently been shown to be a normal plasma alpha globulin.

It was originally believed that these protein structures were embedded in a mucopolysaccharide matrix, but it is now more likely that amyloid is composed purely of protein.

Glenner et al (1968) has isolated the amyloid fibrils and has examined their physical properties and amino-acid sequences. His results indicate that amyloid is composed of light-chain polypeptides arranged in a β-pleated sheeted pattern.

The diagnosis of amyloid

Since the virtual disappearance of the intravenous Congo red test the diagnosis of amyloidosis has been based on the histological demonstration of amyloid in biopsy specimens.

Numerous biopsy sites have been proposed but the best sites are rectum, gingiva and kidney. Of these, *rectal biopsy* is the method of choice in the majority of cases. Providing the biopsy specimen is adequate (in other words, contains enough submucosa to provide a reasonable number of small arterioles in the walls of which amyloid can be sought), rectal biopsy gives a high detection rate in all types of systematised amyloidosis. The biopsy is easily and quickly performed, and is a painless, safe procedure.

Of course, if the patient has manifestations of possible renal involvement renal biopsy is theoretically the best diagnostic manoeuvre. However, since the technique is not without risk it is probably best performed only in renal units where renal biopsies are an everyday procedure, or by a clinician with considerable renal biopsy experience. Otherwise rectal biopsy is preferable.

Gingival biopsy has no real advantage over rectal biopsy, is more painful, and gives a lower detection rate.

DEMONSTRATION OF AMYLOID

Preparation of tissue

In our experience, it is considerably easier to demonstrate all types of amyloid in fresh frozen sections than in paraffin sections. All the standard amyloid staining techniques are more successful on cryostat sections, the methyl violet being the most remarkable in this respect in that the smallest concentrations of methyl violet will colour amyloid bright pink whilst leaving the background clear. In the majority of cases, however, there is no alternative to the use of paraffin sections; in these circumstances it appears that a short fixation will give a better result than overfixation. The choice of fixative does not appear to be critical and satisfactory results are obtained with formol saline.

Staining of amyloid

POSTMORTEM ROOM

Amyloid can be demonstrated on fresh tissues by treatment with iodine and potassium iodide. The deposit is stained a nutmeg-brown colour, which changes to blue-violet by treatment with dilute sulphuric acid.

HISTOLOGY LABORATORY

A considerable number of methods, with various modifications, are available to demonstrate amyloid. However, there is no single method that is specific for amyloid alone; electron microscopy is the only technique at present which can fulfil that role. The existing histological methods in routine use fall into three categories: congo red type (Congo red, Sirius red), metachromatic (methyl violet, crystal violet), and fluorescent (thioflavine T, acridine yellow, Congo red).

Congo red type

The technique, first introduced by Bennhold (1922), stains amyloid deposits an orange to red colour (Fig. 5.1a). There are many variations of the method and in our hands the best two are those of Highman (1946), and the alkaline Congo red technique of Puchtler, Sweat and Levene (1962). In the standard Congo red methods staining occurs when the section is overstained in Congo red and then differentiated, as amyloid has a greater affinity for Congo red than most other tissues. Differentiation is carried out until the Congo red stain has been removed from most other tissue elements but remains in the amyloid deposits. This technique calls for accurate differentiation for if too little of the excess stain is removed then structures other than amyloid will appear positive, e.g. hyaline and collagen. If too much stain is removed then true amyloid deposits are missed.

The alkaline Congo red method (Puchtler et al, 1962) avoids this danger in that it needs no differentiation. It is, however, time-consuming and more difficult to use and occasionally, due to the alkalinity of the solution, sections tend to become detached from the slide. One of the disadvantages of the Congo red methods is that the orange-red colour produced is, under the best conditions, only of moderate intensity, particularly with the alkaline method. The major advantage of the Congo red technique is that amyloid stained with Congo red and viewed by polarised light exhibits characteristic positive apple-green birefringence (Fig. 5.1b).

Metachromatic stains

This type of method employs either methyl or crystal violet. There is some debate as to whether the pink-staining metachromasia, obtained when using methyl violet on deposits of amyloid, is true metachromasia. Methyl violet is a triphenylmethane dye and is a mixture of tetra-, penta- and hexa-methyl pararosaniline. Since the dye is a mixture its staining characteristics may be due to a selective staining by one of the coloured components of the dye mixture and not true metachromasia.

This technique was the first satisfactory histological method to demonstrate amyloid, but with the development of new techniques the method is little used today due to the failure of some amyloid deposits to stain, and non-specific staining of other substances is sometimes seen.

Toluidine blue can also be used to demonstrate amyloid following partial peptic digestion of amyloid deposits. After partial digestion the staining of the deposits changes from orthochromatic (blue) to metachromatic (red) with either toluidine blue or azure A.

Fluorescent methods

Some tissue components exhibit autofluorescence when viewed with a fluorescence microscope. The autofluorescence of amyloid appears brighter than that exhibited by most tissue elements but not enough to make it a useful technique on its own. Vassar and Culling (1959) did a considerable amount of work comparing many fluorochromes (dyes that have the ability to fluoresce). They recommended thioflavine T as a fluorochrome suitable to demonstrate amyloid. Amyloid deposits fluoresce brilliantly under ultraviolet light with a clarity that surpasses any other type of method to demonstrate amyloid (Fig. 5.1d). It is extremely sensitive and will demonstrate very small deposits, unfortunately it is non-specific in that other structures and tissues may fluoresce (e.g. some hyaline). It is ideal as a scanning method, but should be used in conjunction with other methods for purposes of specific diagnosis of amyloid.

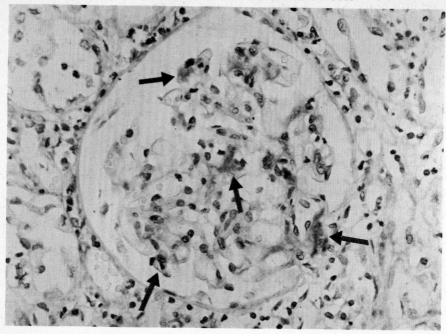

Figure 5.1 (a) A glomerulus, stained with Congo red, showing minimal deposits of amyloid (arrowed). Such small amounts would almost certainly be missed on an H & E stain, and are not very obvious on a Congo red stain. Magnification (× 392)

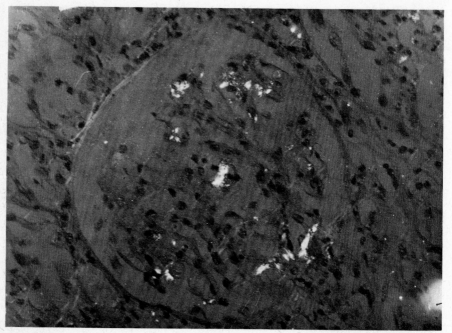

(b) The same glomerulus, again stained with Congo red, but photographed using polarised light. The amyloid deposits stand out by virtue of their birefringence; apple-green dichroism confirms their amyloid nature. Magnification (× 392)

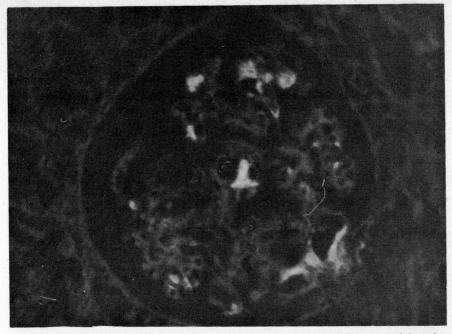

(c) The same glomerulus, this time very lightly stained with Congo red and photographed through a fluorescence microscope. The amyloid deposits show orange-red fluorescence. Magnification (× 392)

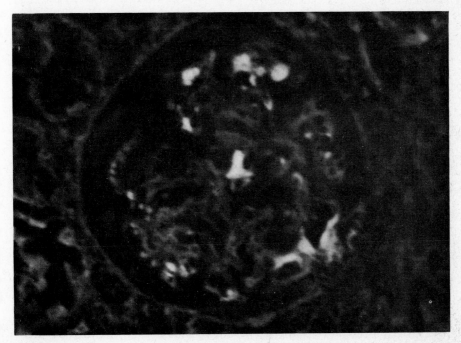

(d) The same glomerulus, stained with thioflavine T and photographed through a fluorescence microscope. The amyloid deposits fluoresce brightly. The fluorescence is more intense than with the Congo red stain, but is less specific. Magnification (× 392)

Other fluorescent dyes may be used to demonstrate amyloid, e.g. acridine yellow, phosphine 3R, coriphosphine and Congo red. A very lightly stained Congo red which may appear negative with the light microscope will exhibit considerable fluorescence of any small amounts of amyloid present (Fig. 5.1c). This method is used routinely in this laboratory and possibly warrants further investigation as a routine method for the demonstration of amyloid. It was first described by Cohen, Calkins and Levene (1959) and is applicable to any Congo red staining method, although we find the best results are obtained with a lightly stained and over-differentiated section that appears negative by the light microscope.

Choice of method

None of the methods described give a constant result with different cases of amyloid. The age of the deposit and the disease with which it is associated appear to be factors involved in this staining variability. In the authors' hands 'primary' amyloid is much more difficult to demonstrate histologically than that associated with other diseases, although both appear identical with the electron microscope. In some cases of experimentally induced amyloid, none of the histological methods prove positive, whilst again the electron microscope showed the characteristic ultrastructural appearances (Fig. 5.2).

Each staining method has its own advantages and disadvantages. The Congo red stain when followed by polarisation is highly specific but possibly a little insensitive, whilst the fluorescent method using thioflavine T tends to be highly sensitive but unfortunately on occasions rather nonspecific. The

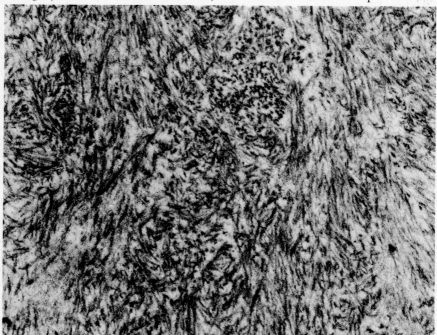

Figure 5.2 Electron micrograph showing the characteristic ultrastructural features of amyloid fibrils. Although the arrangement of the fibrils is largely haphazard, there is some tendency for them to be clumped in groups. In the centre of the picture some of the clumps have been cut transversely. From a skin biopsy of a patient with amyloid in the skin. Magnification ($\times$ 34,996)

metachromatic techniques using methyl or crystal violet are non-specific. In practice amyloid should not be diagnosed on one technique alone; at least two methods should be used, one of which should be a Congo red technique followed by polarisation.

OPTICAL METHODS

Until the advent of the electron microscope, the polarising microscope played a very significant role in the studies of the submicroscopic structure of tissue and cells. The first indication that amyloid might have an organised periodic structure was obtained using a polarising microscope by Divry and Florkin (1927). Today polarisation is used in conjunction with the Congo red method to confirm the presence of amyloid; amyloid in an unstained state or stained by haematoxylin and eosin will exhibit a weak yellow birefringence, but an amyloid deposit stained with Congo red will exhibit positive apple-green birefringence.

Positive apple-green birefringence with Congo red is also seen with certain plant substances and artificially created proteins, the common feature of both groups being a beta-pleated sheet pattern. Note that some collagen and bowel may occasionally show apple-green birefringence.

A summary of amyloid-staining methods is given in Table 5.1.

Table 5.1. Amyloid-staining methods

Method	Results	Comment
Haematoxylin and eosin	Amorphous pink deposit	Easily missed with small deposits
Methyl/crystal violet	Metachromatic pink; purple in paraffin sections	Technically unsatisfactory; non-specific staining occurs
Congo red	Orange-red	Best available; when followed by dichroism is most specific method; also fluorescent
Sirius red	Orange-red	No advantage over Congo red
Periodic acid Schiff	Pale pink or negative	No diagnostic use, results vary with deposit
Thioflavine T	Bright fluorescence, colour depends upon filters and wavelength	Excellent scanning method; very sensitive, but non-specific; always use with another method
Pepsin digestion (see Bancroft, 1975)	Pale pink if eosin used	Specific but technically difficult
DMAB for protein★ (see Bancroft, 1975)	Blue	Positive for amyloid but not specific
Van Gieson	Khaki	Can be used for scanning; not specific; no diagnostic use

★ The DMAB method uses *p*-dimethyl aminobenzaldehyde in acid solution, followed by sodium nitrite to demonstrate tryptophan.

STAINING METHODS
Methyl violet method for amyloid

METHOD
1. Place sections in xylol, then down to water.
2. Stain in 0.5 per cent methyl violet for 2 minutes.

E

3. Wash in water.
4. Examine under the microscope, differentiate in 0.1 per cent acetic acid until amyloid is purple-red.
5. Wash in tap water.
6. Place in saturated solution of sodium chloride for 5 minutes. (See note 1.)
7. Wash in tap water.
8. Mount in Apathy's medium.

RESULTS
Amyloid: *purple-red* to *red.*
Nuclei: *blue.*
Background: *blue.*

NOTES
1. In the screening of surgical material, i.e. rectal biopsies, it is recommended that the pathologist or an experienced technologist looks at the slide at this stage as well as after mounting.
2. The dye will slowly leak out into the mounting medium, so the slides will deteriorate with time.

Congo red (Highman 1946)
   This method is probably the best of the standard Congo red techniques and, with accurate differentiation is highly selective. Polarisation should be used to confirm that the deposit is amyloid (i.e. shows apple-green birefringence.)

METHOD
1. Place sections in xylol, then down to water.
2. Stain in 0.5 per cent Congo red in 50 per cent alcohol for 5 minutes.
3. Wash in water.
4. Differentiate in 0.2 per cent potassium hydroxide in 80 per cent alcohol for 1–2 minutes; this must be controlled microscopically.
5. Wash in water.
6. Counterstain in haematoxylin for 5 minutes.
7. Wash in water.
8. Dehydrate, clear and mount.

RESULTS
Amyloid: *orange-red.*
Nuclei: *blue.*

NOTES
Differentiation is critical and experience is needed to avoid false positives or negatives.

Alkaline Congo red method (Puchtler et al, 1962)
   A recent modification of the Congo red method is considered to be more selective and does not require differentiation. It is, however, more time-consuming and difficult to use than the previous method. For confirmation of amyloid deposits polarisation must be employed as with other Congo red methods.

SOLUTIONS

Alkaline solution
  (a) Stock solution: 80 per cent alcohol saturated with sodium chloride.
  (b) Working solution: add 0.5 ml of 1 per cent sodium hydroxide (aqueous) to 50 ml of stock solution. Filter and use immediately.

Congo red solution
  (a) Stock solution: 80 per cent alcohol saturated with sodium chloride and Congo red.
  (b) Working solution: add 0.5 ml 1 per cent sodium hydroxide (aqueous) to 50 ml of stock solution. Filter and use immediately.

METHOD
  1. Place sections in xylol, then down to water.
  2. Stain nuclei in alum haematoxylin.
  3. Wash in water.
  4. Differentiate in 1 per cent acid alcohol.
  5. Treat with alkaline solution for 20 minutes.
  6. Stain in Congo red solution for 20 minutes.
  7. Rinse in absolute alcohol.
  8. Rinse in fresh absolute alcohol.
  9. Place in xylol.
 10. Mount in DPX.

RESULTS
Amyloid: *pink to red.*
Nuclei: *blue.*
Elastic fibres: *pink.*

NOTES
  1. The Congo red stock solution should stand overnight before being used.
  2. This technique may be used as a fluorescent method.

Congo red method for fluorescence (Cohen et al, 1959; Puchtler and Sweat, 1965)

METHOD
  1. Place sections in xylol, then down to water.
  2. Stain in 0.1 per cent Congo red in 50 per cent alcohol for 1 minute.
  3. Wash in tap water.
  4. Differentiate in 0.2 per cent potassium hydroxide in 80 per cent alcohol until all colour is out of the section.
  5. Wash in water.
  6. Dehydrate through clean alcohols to fresh xylol and mount in fluorescence-free mountant, or after stage 5 mount in Apathy's medium.

RESULTS
  Under the fluorescence microscope amyloid deposits fluoresce orange to red.

NOTES
1. Small deposits of amyloid are shown well by this method.
2. In certain situations especially bowel biopsy specimens, occasional cells, possibly argyrophil cells, show fluorescence.
3. The alkaline Congo red method given previously may also be used.

Thioflavine T fluorescent method (Vassar and Culling, 1959)

METHOD
1. Place sections in xylol, then down to water.
2. Stain in haematoxylin (Mayer's) for 3 minutes.
3. Wash in tap water.
4. Stain in filtered 1 per cent thioflavine T (aqueous) for 3 minutes.
5. Rinse in water.
6. Remove excess staining with 1 per cent acetic acid for 20 minutes.
7. Wash well in water.
8. Dehydrate through *clean* graded alcohols to fresh xylol.
9. Mount in a fluorescence-free mountant, or following stage 7 mount in Apathy's medium.

RESULTS
Amyloid: *bright yellow*.
This colour can be changed by using different filters.

NOTES
1. Maximum fluorescence is not seen immediately after staining.
2. Eosin contaminating the dehydrating alcohols will cause pink fluorescence.
3. Thioflavine T solution should be kept in a dark bottle. Fresh solution should be prepared at 3-month intervals.
4. Non-specific autofluorescence of tissues containing no amyloid should always be considered.
5. In certain situations, especially bowel biopsy specimens, occasional cells, possibly argyrophil cells, show fluorescence.

REFERENCES

BANCROFT, J. D. (1975). *An Introduction to Histochemical Technique*, 2nd edition. London: Butterworths (in Press).
BENNHOLD, H. (1922). Eine spezipische amyloidfarbung mit Kongorot. *Munchen med. Wschr.*, **69**, 1537.
COHEN, A. S. (1967). Amyloidosis. *New Engl. J. Med.*, **227**, 523.
COHEN, A. S., CALKINS, E. & LEVENE, C. (1959). Analysis of histology and staining reactions of casein induced amyloidosis in the rabbit. *Amer. J. Path.*, **35**, 971.
DIVRY, P. & FLORKIN, M. (1927). Sur les proprietes optiques de l'amyloide. *C.R. Soc. Biol. (Paris)*, **97**, 1808.
GLENNER, G. G., KEISER, H. R., BLADDEN, H. A., CUATRECASAS, P., EANES, E. D., RAM, J. S., KANFER, J. N. & DeLELLIS, R. A. (1968). Amyloid 4. A comparison of two morphologic components of human amyloid deposits. *J. Histochem. Cytochem.*, **16**, 633.
HIGHMAN, B. (1946). Improved methods for demonstrating amyloid in paraffin sections. *Arch. Path.*, **41**, 559.
PUCHTLER, H. & SWEAT, F. (1965). Congo red as a stain for fluorescence microscopy of amyloid. *J. Histochem. Cytochem.*, **13**, 693.
PUCHTLER, H., SWEAT, F. & LEVENE, M. (1962). On the binding of Congo red by amyloid. *J. Histochem. Cytochem.*, **10**, 355.
VASSAR, P. S. & CULLING, C. F. A. (1959). Fluorescent stains, with especial reference to amyloid and connective tissue. *Arch. Path.*, **68**, 487.

FURTHER READING

COHEN, A. S. & CALKINS, E. (1959). Electron microscopic observations on a fibrous component in amyloid of diverse origins. *Nature*, **183**, 1202.

COHEN, A. S. (1967). Amyloidosis. *New Engl. J. Med.*, **277**, 522–529, 628–638.

COHEN, A. S. (1971). Trends in clinical and basic amyloid research. *New Engl. J. Med.*, **285**, 576.

FRANCIS, R. (1973). In *Histopathology: Selected Topics*, ed. Cook, H. C. London: Baillière Tindall.

The writings of G. G. GLENNER and co-authors.

GLENNER, G. G., HARADA, M., ISERSKY, C., CUATRECASAS, P., PAGE, D. KEISER, H. (1970). Human amyloid protein: diversity and uniformity. *Biochem. Biophys. Res. Commun.*, **41**, 1013.

GLENNER, G. G., EIN, D., EANES, E. D., BLADEN, H. A., TERRY, W. & PAGE, D. L. (1971). Creation of 'amyloid' fibrils from Bence Jones proteins in vitro. *Science*, **174**, 712.

GLENNER, G. G., TERRY, W., HARADA, M., ISERSKY, C. & PAGE, D. L. (1971). Amyloid fibril proteins: proof of homology with immunoglobulin light chains by sequence analyses. *Science*, **172**, 1150.

GLENNER, G. G., EIN, D. & TERRY, W. D. (1972). The immunoglobulin origin of amyloid. *Amer. J. Med.*, **52**, 141.

PEARSE, A. G. E. (1968). *Histochemistry, Theoretical and Applied*, Vol. 1, pp. 381–398. London: Churchill.

PUCHTLER, H. & SWEAT, F. (1966). A review of early concepts of amyloid in context with contemporary chemical literature from 1839–1859. *J. Histochem. Cytochem.*, **14**, 123.

CHAPTER 6
Central Nervous System

Neuropathology is a specialised branch of histopathology in which only those pathologists and technicians who have access to a lot of material can hope to acquire all-round competence, although all pathologists are able to diagnose the more commonly seen conditions such as brain tumours, infarcts, or disseminated sclerosis.

Fixation of the brain removed at necropsy

Most pathologists fix the brain in toto by suspending it in a large container of formalin by a string attached to the basilar artery; full fixation takes about six to eight weeks, although the brain is usually firm enough to dissect or slice after two to three weeks. Unfortunately the brain is frequently damaged or distorted by the handling during its removal from the skull, particularly if parts of the brain are abnormally soft (e.g. following cerebral infarction or haemorrhage) or abnormally swollen (e.g. in association with cerebral tumours). This can be minimised by partly fixing the brain in situ some time before the necropsy is to be performed.

The following technique has been used by us on a number of occasions when interest has centred on the brain. On the afternoon before the necropsy is to be performed, the neck is opened and the internal carotid artery is cannulated on one side, and opened on the other. Ten per cent formol saline is pumped up the cannulated carotid artery using a simple controllable pressure pumping device such as a mortician's embalming pump. When clear formalin appears at the opened carotid artery on the other side the cannulated carotid is tied off and the opened carotid on the other side is cannulated and a little formalin pumped in before the second carotid is tied off. In the majority of cases the hind brain is adequately perfused in this way without having to cannulate the vertebral artery system. The body is left overnight and the brain removed in the normal manner the following day. By this time the brain is partly fixed and is more rigid; since it is less pliable and manoeuvrable, a little more care is needed when the brain is removed. The brain is then suspended in a container of formalin in the normal manner to complete fixation of the cortex; if the perfusion has been adequate the brain is usually ready for slicing only two or three days after removal. The advantages of perfusing in situ are many: in most cases there is no artefactual distortion or tearing of the brain, the brain can be sliced and examined properly some weeks earlier than if fixed solely by the immersion method, fixative gets quickly to important areas like the internal capsule which are usually the last parts to be fixed by immersion, and the histology is correspondingly much improved.

The technique is simplicity in itself and can be performed by the mortuary attendant.

Fixation of the spinal cord

The spinal cord is carefully removed and suspended vertically in a long tube containing 10 per cent formol saline. Slightly modified used fluorescent light tubes are suitable for this purpose; they can be obtained free of charge in any hospital and are usually available in large numbers. It is advisable to open the ensheathing dura before fixation, either by making careful longitudinal scissor cuts anteriorly and posteriorly, or, less riskily, making a series of nicks in the dura with scissors or a sharp scalpel throughout the length of the cord anteriorly and posteriorly. In this way fixation time can be reduced from two weeks to one week as a maximum.

Processing and embedding of brain and spinal cord tissue

Nervous tissue can be embedded either in paraffin wax, celloidin or low viscosity nitrocellulose. Paraffin wax is suitable for small pieces, although it must be said that double embedding using low viscosity nitrocellulose (which has largely replaced celloidin) gives technically superior results. We use paraffin wax for urgent material because the low-viscosity nitrocellulose method is time-consuming and processing can take one to two weeks. For a detailed account of double embedding techniques readers are referred to Disbrey and Rack (1970) and Drury and Wallington (1967).

Cells of the central nervous system

The cells found in the central nervous system can be simply divided into three basic types:

Nerve Cells (Neurones)

These are large cells with long and short cytoplasmic processes (nerve fibres, axons) extruded from them. Some of these processes are ensheathed in *myelin*, a lipid and lipoprotein material which is responsible for the 'whiteness' of the white matter in the brain and spinal cord. The neurones are embedded in, and supported and nourished by, tissue known as glial tissue (neuroglia).

Neuroglia

Neuroglial cells can be divided into the following types:

(a) *Astrocytes*. These supporting cells exist in two recognised forms, protoplasmic astrocytes and so-called 'fibrous' astrocytes. Protoplasmic astrocytes have short, stout cytoplasmic processes which branch finely at their ends; they occur particularly in the grey matter of the brain. 'Fibrous' astrocytes have very long and fine fibrillary cytoplasmic processes which do not branch as much as those of the protoplasmic astrocytes; they are found particularly in the white matter of the brain and spinal cord, and in smaller numbers in the superficial grey matter of the brain. The types of astrocytes can be best distinguished by special stains which demonstrate the cytoplasmic processes.

(b) *Oligodendroglia*. These cells are present in small numbers and are responsible for the production and maintenance of the myelin sheaths around nerve fibres.

(c) *Microglia*. Microglial cells are small and resemble lymphocytes and may serve a similar function; they are widely regarded as a specialised component of the reticulo-endothelial system, rather than true neuroglial cells.

EPENDYMA

The ventricles of the brain are lined by ependymal cells which have a pseudo-epithelial appearance. They can be shown to have cilia which presumably assist in the circulation of cerebrospinal fluid. Ependymal cells play very little part in pathological processes in the brain.

Staining

The routine stain for use with brain and spinal cord sections is again the H & E, but this does not adequately demonstrate the fine structure, and nerve fibres and myelin cannot be distinguished. The following methods are commonly used:

1. Haematoxylin and eosin.
2. A stain for nerve fibres (e.g. Glees and Marsland, Holmes).
3. A stain for normal myelin (e.g. Loyez, Weil's short method).
4. A stain for Nissl substance (e.g. cresyl violet).
5. A general stain for neuroglial cells and fibres (PTAH).

Methods exist for the specific demonstration of astrocytes (Cajal, Hortega) and microglia and oligodendroglia (Weil and Davenport, Rio-Hortega, Penfield). All are gold or silver impregnation methods and must be performed on frozen sections. They tend to be capricious and often prove unreliable as an occasionally performed stain. However, in CNS-orientated laboratories where these methods are used regularly the results are both informative and aesthetically pleasing. Poor results are obtained unless the brain tissue is very fresh; necropsy material is rarely suitable unless removed within 24 hours of death.

STAINS FOR NERVE FIBRES

Most nerve fibre methods are based on silver impregnation and can be performed on paraffin sections. Our preference is for the Glees and Marsland technique (Fig. 6.1). The Holmes technique gives just as good results but is more time-consuming and for the best result microscopic control is needed.

STAINS FOR NORMAL MYELIN

The most widely used methods for normal myelin are based on the fact that myelin is stained by haematoxylins after suitable iron mordanting. Our preference is for a variant of the Loyez method; in the Loyez method the tissue section is mordanted in 4 per cent iron alum for 24 hours before staining with haematoxylin and subsequent differentiation. *Weil's modification* is basically similar and the technique can be completed within an hour; in this method the mordant (iron alum) is mixed with the haematoxylin and the tissue mordanted and stained at the same time at 45–50°C for 15 minutes. This short method has proved highly satisfactory in our hands and the results are in no way inferior to those obtained by the longer Loyez method (Figs. 6.2a, b).

When myelin degenerates after trauma or other damage the complex lipid–lipoprotein mixture breaks down to release, amongst other things, a mixture of fatty acids and simple fats. By virtue of the simple fats produced, degenerating myelin can be demonstrated by simple lipid stains (e.g. oil red O) on frozen sections. A more time-consuming (4–7 days) method is that of Marchi, which is based on the blackening of oleic acid (produced by the breakdown

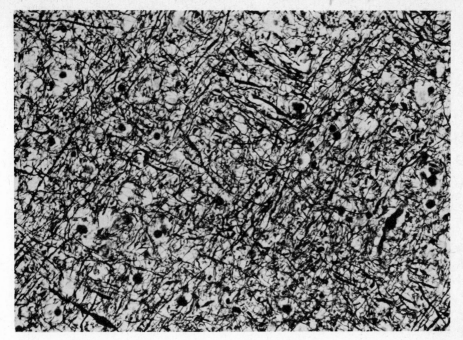

Figure 6.1 Brain stained by the Glees and Marsland silver method to demonstrate nerve fibres. Glees and Marsland (× 420)

of myelin) by osmium tetroxide. Degenerate myelin can usually only be demonstrated from about 10 days to 12 weeks after tissue damage.

STAINS FOR NISSL SUBSTANCE

Nissl substance is found in the cytoplasm of healthy neurones and can be demonstrated using the cresyl violet stain. All the tissue initially takes up the stain, but the stain is washed out with 96 per cent alcohol until only the Nissl substance in the nerve cells retains the purple colour (Fig. 6.3). If the differentiation with alcohol is stopped before the stage at which only Nissl substance is purple, the cresyl violet stain is a good method to demonstrate the general cellular structure of the nervous system. Nissl substance can also be demonstrated by other techniques including the Unna–Pappenheim method (methyl green pyronin).

The importance of Nissl substance to the pathologist lies in its being a very sensitive indicator of nerve cell damage. When neurones suffer irreversible damage the Nissl substance within them disappears and the neurones later degenerate.

THE PTAH STAIN FOR NEUROGLIA

Mallory's PTAH stain is a useful stain for demonstrating the astrocytic reaction to tissue damage in the CNS; it stains glial cells and fibres blue. Holzer's method, though rather intricate, is specific for glial fibres.

Frozen sections

Frozen sections are essential:

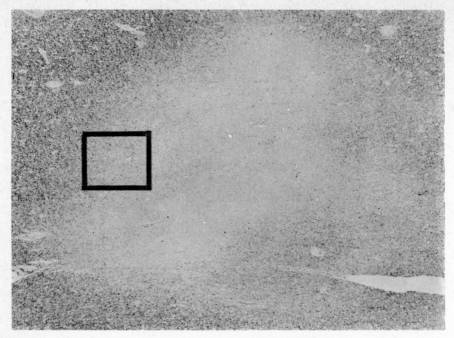

Figure 6.2 (a) Brain stained by Weil's short method for myelin. A pale-staining area of demyelination can be seen. The patient had disseminated sclerosis. Magnification (× 40)

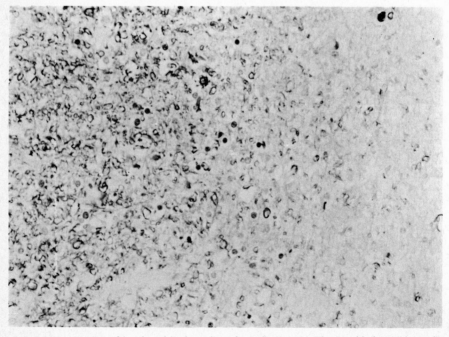

(b) High power view of the edge of the demyelinated area shown in (a). The grey-black staining myelin sheaths can easily be seen in the more normal area of the brain. They are virtually absent from the demyelinated area. Weil's stain for myelin. Magnification (× 392)

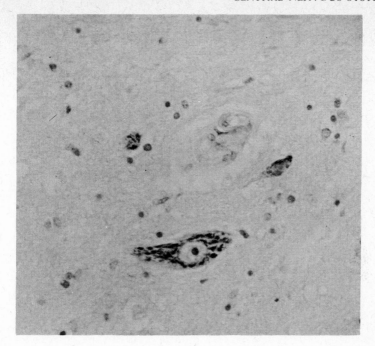

Figure 6.3 A Nissl stain (cresyl violet) showing the Nissl substance in a normal neurone. Magnification (× 392)

(a) for rapid diagnosis of biopsy material, e.g. brain tumours. A rapid H & E is usually all that is required,
(b) for the demonstration of fat (e.g. fat embolism in postmortem brain, or to demonstrate degenerate myelin). The oil red O stain is the most satisfactory,
(c) for the successful demonstration of astrocytes, microglia and oligo-dendroglia using the silver and gold impregnation techniques of Cajal, Rio-Hortega, etc,
(d) for the histochemical identification of lipids and lipoproteins of certain so-called 'lipid storage diseases' in the CNS.

Small blocks are preferably cut on a cryostat, although the freezing microtome may be used for larger pieces of tissue.

Electron microscopy

In routine service neuropathology, there is, as yet, little call for electron microscopy of brain or spinal cord; it remains largely a research procedure. Small fragments of fresh tissue are fixed in buffered glutaraldehyde, osmium tetroxide and embedded in araldite. Sections are cut on the ultratome in the normal manner; sections can also be cut at 1μ on the ultratome or pyramitome and stained by toluidine blue stain.

A summary of staining techniques is given in Table 6.1.

Table 6.1. Standard techniques for the central nervous system

Staining method	Demonstrates	Type of section	Page
Bielschowski's	Nerve endings	Frozen	—
Glees and Marsland, Holmes, Bodian	Nerve fibres	Paraffin	68
PTAH	Neuroglia cells and fibres	Paraffin	8
Holzer's	Glial fibres	Any	—
Hortega's, Cajal's	Astrocytes	Frozen	—
Weil, Davenport	Microglia, oligodendroglia	Frozen, paraffin	—
Rio–Hortega's, Penfield	Microglia, oligodendroglia	Frozen	—
Weil	Normal myelin	Any	66
Loyez, Weigert, Pal	Normal myelin	Paraffin celloidin	—
Marchi	Degenerate myelin	Paraffin celloidin	—
Swank–Davenport	Degenerate myelin	Frozen	67
Oil red O	Lipids, degenerate myelin	Frozen	32
Unna—Pappenheim	Nissl granules	Paraffin	—
Gallocyanin, toluidine blue			
Cresyl fast violet	Nissl granules	Any	67

STAINING METHODS

Weil's technique for normal myelin (Weil, 1928, modified)

This is a rapid method, which is a modification of the Loyez technique. In our hands it works well and is used routinely. Thick sections 15–20 μ should be used.

Weil's haematoxylin

10 per cent haematoxylin in absolute alcohol	5 ml
4 per cent iron alum	50 ml
Distilled water	45 ml

Weigert's differentiating fluid

Sodium tetraborate	2 g
Potassium ferricyanide	2.5 g
Distilled water	200 ml

METHOD
1. Place paraffin sections in xylol, then down to water.
2. Rinse in distilled water.
3. Stain in Weil's haematoxylin at 37°C for 30 minutes.
4. Wash in tap water for 30 minutes.
5. Differentiate in 4 per cent iron alum.
6. Wash in tap water for 5 minutes.
7. Complete differentiation in Weigert's fluid.
8. Wash in tap water.
9. Dehydrate, clear and mount in DPX.

RESULTS
Myelin: *blue–black*.
Background: *pale grey*.

NOTES
1. Differentiate in iron alum (step 5) until there is a distinct difference between white and grey matter.
2. In the differentiation with Weigert's fluid, look particularly at the area at the junction between white and grey matter to pick up myelinated (grey–black) fibres penetrating a little way into the more palely staining grey matter.

Cresyl fast violet method for Nissl granules

SOLUTIONS
Cresyl fast violet

Cresyl fast violet	0.1 g
Distilled water	99 ml
1 per cent acetic acid	1 ml

METHOD
1. Place sections in xylol, then down to water.
2. Stain sections in cresyl fast violet solution at 60°C for 1–10 minutes.
3. Differentiate in 96 per cent alcohol under microscopic control (see note 1).
4. Rinse in absolute alcohol.
5. Clear and mount in DPX.

RESULTS
Nissl granules: *violet*.
Nuclei: *pale violet*.

NOTES
1. Different staining times are required according to how the tissue has been prepared: frozen sections, 1–4 minutes; celloidin, 3–5 minutes; paraffin, 5–10 minutes.
2. The staining solution does not keep well.
3. Some batches of dye will fail to work.

Swank–Davenport method for degenerate myelin (Swank and Davenport, 1935)

This method is a modification of the Marchi technique to demonstrate degenerate myelin. The method is applied to 50μ thick frozen sections.

SOLUTION
Marchi's solution

1 per cent potassium chlorate	60 ml
1 per cent osmium tetroxide	20 ml
Formalin	12 ml
Glacial acetic acid	1 ml

METHOD
1. Fix tissue in 10 per cent formol saline.
2. Cut frozen sections 40–50 μ thick.
3. Leave in Marchi's solution for 5–7 days.
4. Wash in distilled water.
5. Mount in glycerin jelly.

RESULT
Degenerate myelin: *black*.

Glees and Marsland technique for nerve fibres (Marsland, Glees and Erikson, 1954)
   This technique is a modification which can be applied to paraffin sections 7 or 8 μ thick.

SOLUTION
Glees silver solution

20 per cent silver nitrate	30 ml
Absolute alcohol	20 ml
Ammonia (.880)	

To the silver nitrate add the absolute alcohol. Add ammonia drop by drop until the first formed precipitate is dissolved. Add a further 4 drops of ammonia.

METHOD
 1. Place sections in xylol, then to absolute alcohol.
 2. Celloidinise, then down to water.
 3. Treat with 20 per cent aqueous silver nitrate solution preheated to 37°C for 30 minutes (section should be yellow-brown).
 4. Wash in 10 per cent formalin until solution runs clear.
 5. Place in fresh 10 per cent formalin for 10 seconds.
 6. Rinse in Glees silver solution rapidly.
 7. Place in Glees silver solution for 30 seconds.
 8. Drain off Glees silver solution.
 9. Wash in 10 per cent formalin for 1 minute.
10. Repeat wash in 10 per cent formalin for 1 minute.
11. Rinse in distilled water.
12. Place in 5 per cent sodium thiosulphate for 2 minutes.
13. Wash well in tap water.
14. Dehydrate, remove celloidin film and any silver precipitate with alcohol ether. Clear and mount in DPX.

RESULTS
Nerve fibres: *black*.

NOTES
1. Examine section under microscope after stage 9. If impregnation is insufficient repeat from stage 6.
2. Toning may be used after stage 11 if required.

REFERENCES

DISBREY, B. D. & RACK, J. H. (1970). *Histological Laboratory Methods.* Edinburgh & London: Livingstone.

DRURY, R. A. B. & WALLINGTON, E. A. (1967). *Carleton's Histological Technique*, 4th edition. London: Oxford University Press.

MARSLAND, T. A., GLEES, P. & ERIKSON, L. B. (1954). Modification of the Glees silver impregnation for paraffin sections. *J. Neuropath. exp. Neurol.,* **13,** 587.

SWANK, R. L. & DAVENPORT, H. A. (1935). Chlorate-osmic-formalin method for staining degenerating myelin. *Stain Technol.,* **10,** 87.

WEIL, A. (1928). A rapid method for staining myelin sheaths. *Arch. Neurol. Psychiat. (Chicago),* **26,** 392.

FURTHER READING

HUME-ADAM, J. & MILLER, L. (1970). *Nervous System Techniques for the General Pathologist,* Broadsheet No. 73, issued by the Association of Clinical Pathologists, London.

McMENEMEY, W. H. (1966). Cytology of the central nervous system. In *Systemic Pathology,* Vol. 2, pp. 1140–1155, by Payling-Wright, G. & Symmers, W. St C. London: Longmans, Green.

SMITH, H. M. & BEESLEY, R. A. (1970). *Practical Neuropathology* (Laboratory Aid Series), ed. Baker, F. J. London: Butterworths.

CHAPTER 7

Calcified and Undecalcified Bone

Bone is a complex tissue composed of an organic matrix, osteoid, in which inorganic calcium salts are deposited in the form of hydroxyapatite crystals.

The *osteoid* is composed largely of proteinaceous fibres (almost certainly collagenous) arranged compactly, together with a mixture of mucopolysaccharides.

The *bone salts* are a crystalline hydroxyapatite composed largely of hydrated calcium phosphate, but also containing traces of carbonate, citrate and other ions. Mineralisation of the osteoid by these bone salts takes place very shortly after the osteoid has been produced by the osteoblasts.

Bone also has a cellular component, there being three important types of cells: the osteoblast, the osteoclast and the osteocyte.

The *osteoblast* is a large polygonal cell, often arranged in neat rows along the edge of a bone trabeculum. Their function seems to be the production of osteoid.

The *osteoclast* is a large, sometimes very large, multinucleate giant cell found at sites of bone erosion or resorption. The more active the bone resorption the larger the osteoclasts seem to be. The mechanism by which osteoclasts erode bone is not fully understood.

The *osteocyte* is generally considered to be an osteoblast which has become trapped within the bone that it has helped to produce.

All bones in the body have, to a greater or lesser extent, two distinct structurally different components, compact bone and loose cancellous bone.

The *compact bone* forms the dense outer shell of bones, and is composed of closely packed cylinders of dense bone with a central canal and containing concentrically arranged osteocytes with cytoplasmic processes running along narrow channels within the bone (canaliculi) and the Haversian canal system.

Cancellous bone is composed of narrow interconnecting trabeculae of bone forming a fine network which has both strength and lightness. This type of pattern forms the central area of a bone and is surrounded by the dense compact, or cortical, bone.

Fixation of bone

As with soft tissues, the adequate fixation of bone is of prime importance. Many fixatives have been tried with bone but the best results are obtained with 10 per cent neutral formol saline. The poor penetration of the fixative is even more of a problem with bone because of the density of the tissue. The average histology block should be fixed for 48 hours and be no thicker than 4 mm to obtain reasonably rapid and good fixation. Some fixatives also contain agents which will decalcify the tissue during fixation; in our experience these produce no better, and often inferior, results than fixation followed by decalcification.

Urgent specimens. Most routine surgical laboratories receive urgent bone biopsies; in these instances fixation must be as rapid as possible. To this end the block selected should be only 2–3 mm thick and fixed in formol saline at 37°C for 4–6 hours with as little cortical or dense bone as possible in the block.

Decalcification or Demineralisation

The hydroxyapatite crystals must be removed from the bone before suitable histology sections can be produced. The removal of these calcium salts is termed *decalcification* or *demineralisation*. To remove the crystals the decalcifying agent must pass through the organic fraction of the tissue before reaching the inorganic fraction, and in doing so invariably damages these structures.

TYPES OF DECALCIFYING AGENT

Two types of reagent may be used for decalcifying, either acids or organic chelating agents.

Acids

Many different acids have been used for decalcifying bone. The acids are used as simple dilute aqueous solutions or in mixed solutions with other dilute acids or chemicals. Out of the many acids the best results are probably obtained with nitric, formic and trichloracetic acids.

Nitric acid. This is probably the most popular of the acids used. It decalcifies rapidly and is reliable in that it will complete the decalcification. Unfortunately, if tissue is left too long in nitric acid considerable damage to the tissue will occur; this damage will become apparent after two days or so at room temperature in concentrations of acid above 8 per cent. Because of its rapid action, nitric acid is ideal for urgent bone biopsies. Nitric acid for routine use should be a 5 per cent solution with a few milligrams of urea added to each 100 ml. After decalcification the tissue is washed well in 70 per cent alcohol before being processed to paraffin wax (Clayden, 1971).

Formic acid. A good routine decalcifying agent, it is slower in its action than nitric acid, but causes less damage to the tissue by overexposure. As a standard reagent it should be used as a 10 per cent solution in distilled water. Decalcification for a piece of cancellous bone 4 mm thick should be complete in 48 hours, while for dense bone two weeks or longer may be required. It is recommended that the formic acid is changed every two days. The staining results obtained after formic acid are superior to those after using nitric acid.

Damage to tissue. Adequate fixation is necessary to minimise the damaging effects of treatment with acids. In using acids to remove calcium ions carbon dioxide is produced; the pressure of the gas and its movement through the tissue is believed to be one of the factors causing the separation of connective tissues seen after decalcification (Brain, 1966). Staining is affected by long treatment with acids in that haematoxylin staining may need to be prolonged and that eosin staining is non-differential and intense.

Chelating agents

Ethylenediamine tetra-acetic acid (EDTA) is the chelating agent used to remove calcium. It produces a much slower rate of decalcification than with acids. The chelation will take place at neutral pH in a 15 per cent solution.

Very little damage occurs to the tissue despite the fact that it may be in the EDTA for several months before decalcification is complete. The speed with which the calcium is removed can be accelerated by slight heat (37°C) without causing tissue damage. Staining is excellent after using this chelating agent and good differential results can be obtained.

Commercial decalcifying agents

These have appeared in recent years; in our hands they have no advantage over laboratory prepared solutions.

Summary

For routine use: 5 per cent nitric acid (aqueous, with added urea) or 10 per cent formic acid (aqueous), 2–4 days.

For non-urgent material: EDTA, 2 weeks–3 months.

For urgent material: warm 5 per cent nitric acid, 5–12 hours.

DETECTING THE END POINT OF DECALCIFICATION

It is important that when decalcification is complete the tissue should be removed from the decalcifying fluid immediately, otherwise damage to the tissue increases and staining is affected. Equally, tissue should remain in the fluid until decalcification is complete, otherwise difficulty will be encountered with cutting. The best way of confirming complete decalcification is to X-ray the specimen; if this facility is not available then a chemical test for the presence of calcium in the decalcifying fluid should be used (see Drury and Wallington, 1967). Once the fluid is free of calcium, decalcification is complete. This test will not work with EDTA as there are no free calcium ions in the decalcifying fluid; in this instance, experience must be used to decide when the specimen is free of calcium if it cannot be X-rayed.

Processing of bone

In handling large pieces of bone consideration must be given after decalcification to how the material is to be embedded. The majority of bone specimens cut adequately when embedded in paraffin wax, in some instances only after double embedding. Dense cortical bone, particularly if a large specimen, will probably give the best results after being embedded in celloidin. Small biopsies of cancellous bone may be processed in the normal way on an overnight schedule.

DOUBLE EMBEDDING PARAFFIN

This is the most suitable technique for producing good sections of bone. It involves the usual dehydration in alcohol, then alcohol–ether, followed by impregnation of the bone in two changes of 2 per cent celloidin. This is followed by hardening of the celloidin and clearing of the tissue, both in chloroform. Finally the block is embedded in paraffin wax, preferably one of the waxes with resin added, such as Fibrowax (R. A. Lamb Ltd, London NW10). This double embedding procedure holds the tissue together better, allowing superior sections to be cut. It takes more time than routine paraffin embedding, usually a working week.

CELLOIDIN SECTIONS

The embedding and sectioning of bone material in celloidin is time-consuming and tedious compared with paraffin wax; it does, however, produce excellent results with large pieces of bone. It is not recommended for routine surgical use.

FROZEN SECTIONS

Small pieces of cancellous bone can be successfully frozen and cut in a cryostat. Larger pieces of bone may be cut on freezing microtomes, but this takes practice before good sections are produced.

Staining of decalcified bone

Unless decalcification with acids has been unnecessarily prolonged, no difficulty should be experienced in staining the sections. The H & E stain is the basic stain for general bone morphology, and very few special stains are required. If decalcification has been in nitric or formic acid, the time in haematoxylin usually needs increasing and the time in eosin reducing. The lamellar and woven patterns of bone are emphasised when an H & E stained section is viewed under crossed polaroids; this is often informative and is always an attractive sight. The van Gieson and trichrome stains for connective tissues may be useful in some tumours or fibrous dysplasias of bone.

Trephine biopsy of bone is sometimes performed by haematologists who are searching for evidence of leukaemic or neoplastic invasion of the bone marrow, or the fibrous replacement of haemopoietic marrow seen in myelofibrosis. The cortical (or compact) bone should be removed from the end of the core and the cancellous bone only is processed for the quickest results. Neoplastic or severe fibrous replacement of the marrow is easily diagnosed on H & E, but marginal fibrous increase may need emphasising by a *reticulin stain*.

Undecalcified bone sections

To investigate the extent of mineralisation of bone, it is necessary to examine undecalcified sections of bone (almost always cancellous bone). Two methods are available for demonstrating the presence of calcium salts: (i) *von Kossa's* technique in which silver is deposited in the calcium, staining mineralised bone black and leaving osteoid unstained to take up the red counterstain, and (ii) *alizarin red S* method in which a stable orange-red lake is formed between the dye and any calcium, osteoid being unstained.

In osteomalacia there is a failure of mineralisation of bone, best seen in the cancellous bone trabeculae; only the central core of the bone is mineralised, the remainder being uncalcified osteoid (Fig. 7.1a). This is distinct from osteoporosis in which although the trabeculae are thin, mineralisation is complete, so no unstained outer zone of osteoid can be distinguished (Fig. 7.1b).

METHOD OF PRODUCTION

Whichever technique is to be used, adequate fixation must first be attained in 10 per cent *neutral* formal saline. A number of techniques are available for producing these sections notably:
(a) sawing and grinding,

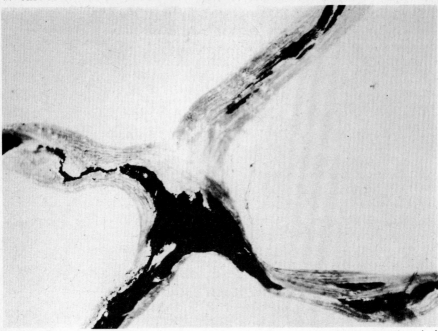

Figure 7.1 (a) An undecalcified resin-embedded section of cancellous bone, stained by von Kossa's method for calcium, from a patient with osteomalacia. The trabeculae are of about normal thickness but only a central narrow core is calcified (stained black); the remainder is non-staining demineralised osteoid. Compare with (b). Magnification ($\times$ 392)

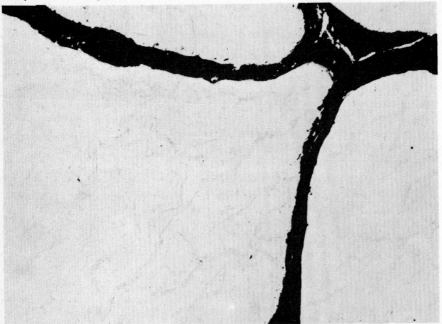

(b) An undecalcified resin-embedded section of cancellous bone, stained by von Kossa's method for calcium, from a patient with osteoporosis. The trabeculae are markedly thinned, although they are totally mineralised. Compare with (a). Magnification ($\times$ 392)

(b) paraffin wax double embedded—using adhesive or gum strip,
(c) resin embedded.

The methods have been used and developed in the order above with a consequent improvement in section quality each time. In our laboratory the undecalcified bone biopsy is embedded in resin as a matter of routine and sections are cut on a Jung K microtome; details of the method are given at the end of the chapter.

A summary of the staining methods for bone is given in Table 7.1.

Table 7.1. Staining methods for use with bone

Method	Application	Page
Haematoxylin and eosin	Morphology	7
van Gieson	Connective tissue	40
Reticulin	Myelofibrosis of bone marrow	41
Periodic acid Schiff	Mucosubstances; woven bone	19
Schmorl thionin★	Lacunae and canaliculi	—
Von Kossa	Calcium deposits (undecalcified bone)	77
Alizarin red S	Calcium deposits (undecalcified bone)	76
Masson's trichrome	Connective tissue	42

★ Not recommended for paraffin sections.

STAINING METHODS

Synthetic resin technique for undecalcified bone

SOLUTIONS
Solution A

Methyl methacrylate monomer	100 ml	(see below)
Benzoyl peroxide	1 g	(see below)
N,N-Butoxyethanol	1 ml	

The inhibitor must be removed from the methyl methacrylate in the following manner:

Place 300 ml of methyl methacrylate monomer in a separating funnel, add 25 ml 5 per cent sodium hydroxide and shake well. Allow sodium hydroxide to settle down then run off, repeat three times or till sodium hydroxide is clear. The excess sodium hydroxide must be removed by adding 50 ml of distilled water and shaking, removing and then repeating three times. It is advisable to dry the methyl methacrylate over anhydrous calcium sulphate overnight.

Benzoyl peroxide on purchase contains 40 per cent water. Dry off in an incubator at 37°C before weighing.

Solution B (partially polymerised methyl methacrylate)

Place 100 ml of solution A in a beaker and heat to 80°C in a water bath. Stir the solution continuously until the solution begins to go viscous. Cool under cold running tap water and store until required at 4°C.

METHOD

The following technique should be followed rigidly, as deviation may result in loss of the biopsy specimen.
1. Fix in 10 per cent *neutral* formol saline for 24 hours.
2. Dehydrate through graded alcohols to absolute alcohol for 2½ days.
3. Degrease in trichlorethylene for 24 hours.
4. Wash in absolute alcohol for 3 hours.
5. Impregnate in solution A at 4°C, 4–7 days with two changes of solution.
6. Place tissue in partially polymerised solution B in a suitable container to make the embedding mould i.e. thin glass-walled test tube (see note 1), at 37°C overnight. When hard remove from mould and trim to suitable size with a small hacksaw.
7. Cut sections at 4–6 μ on Jung K microtome, moistening the block with 70 per cent alcohol.
8. Place cut sections into 70 per cent alcohol.
9. Rinse in distilled water and stain sections free-floating.

NOTES
1. Treat the test tube with a 'non-stick' compound such as Repelcote (Hopkin and Williams Ltd) before use.
2. Sections can be stained by von Kossa, alizarin red S and haematoxylin and eosin.
3. An alternative method to staining sections free-floating is at stage 8 to place the cut sections in a solution of absolute alcohol and butoxyethanol (9:1). The sections are picked up on albuminised slides, clamped between filter paper and another slide with a bulldog clip and dried overnight at 40°C. The following morning the methacrylate is removed by treatment with 2-methoxyethyl acetate. In our experience, however, a percentage of sections float off the slides. For this reason we prefer to use the free-floating sections.

A recent simplified method, involving the slow cold mixing of preformed poly (methyl methacrylate) with catalysed monomer, has been suggested by Difford (1974). In our hands this modification has worked very well and minimises the problems inherent in using heat in the preparation of the resin.

Alizarin red 'S' for calcium deposits (Dahl, 1952; McGee-Russell, 1958)
This method requires a little practice before consistently good results are obtained.

METHOD
1. Place sections in xylol, then down to water.
2. Transfer sections to 2 per cent aqueous alizarin red S stain at pH 4.2 (with 10 per cent NH_4OH) for 1–4 minutes.
3. Blot.
4. Rinse rapidly in distilled water.
5. Blot.
6. Rinse rapidly on 0.1 per cent HCl in 95 per cent alcohol for 10 seconds.
7. Rinse in 95 per cent alcohol.
8. Rinse in absolute alcohol.
9. Clear in xylol and mount in DPX.

RESULTS
Calcium deposits: *orange-red*.

NOTES
   Stage 2 must be controlled microscopically until the staining reaction is strong but not diffuse.

Von Kossa for calcium deposits (von Kossa, 1901)
   This method can be employed for free-floating resin-embedded material and for conventional paraffin sections. Resin sections should be transferred direct to stage 2.

METHOD
1. Place sections in xylol, then down to water.
2. Wash well in distilled water for 3–5 minutes.
3. Place in 2 per cent silver nitrate (see note below).
4. Wash well in distilled water for 3 minutes.
5. Place in 5 per cent sodium thiosulphate for 2 minutes.
6. Wash well in distilled water.
7. Counterstain in 1 per cent neutral red for 1 minute (see note 2).
8. Rinse rapidly in tap water.
9. Dehydrate rapidly, clear and mount in DPX.

RESULTS
Calcium deposits: *brown-black*.
Nuclei: *red*.

NOTES
1. The time in the silver solution depends upon exposure. If the sections in the solution are exposed to ultraviolet light, 5 minutes is long enough. Exposure to strong daylight takes 30–60 minutes. Exposure to strong artificial light requires approximately 1 hour.
2. When used with undecalcified bone sections, best results are obtained with a van Gieson counterstain. The osteoid stains bright red with the acid fuchsin.

REFERENCES
BRAIN, E. B. (1966). *The Preparation of Decalcified Sections.* Springfield, Illinois: Thomas.
CLAYDEN, E. C. (1971). *Practical Section Cutting and Staining,* 5th edition. Edinburgh & London: Churchill Livingstone.
DAHL, L. K. (1952). Simple and sensitive histochemical method for calcium. *Proc. Soc. exp. Biol. (N.Y.),* **80,** 474.
DIFFORD, J. (1974). A simplified method for the preparation of methyl methacrylate embedding medium for undecalcified bone. *Medical Laboratory Technology,* **31,** 79.
DRURY, R. A. B. & WALLINGTON, E. A. (1967). *Carleton's Histological Technique,* 4th edition. London: Oxford University Press.
KOSSA, J. VON (1901). Ueber die im organismus Kunstlich eizugberen verkalkungen. *Beitr. path. Anat.,* **29,** Suppl. iv, 163.
MCGEE-RUSSELL, S. M. (1958). Histochemical methods for calcium. *J. Histochem. Cytochem.,* **6,** 22.

FURTHER READING

WALLINGTON, E. A. (1972). *Histological Methods for Bone* (Laboratory Aids Series) ed. Baker, F. J. London: Butterworths.

SISSONS, H. A. (1968). *Preparation of Undecalcified Bone Sections*, Broadsheet No. 62. Issued by the Association of Clinical Pathologists, London.

CHAPTER 8
Pigments and Metals

A wide variety of pigments may be found in histological sections; some are *artefactual* deposits, the result of an interaction between a tissue component and some component of the fixative. Many pigments are *autogenous*, being normal products of cellular metabolism, although they may be produced in excessive amounts or deposited in unusual sites in certain pathological states. Some *exogenous* materials may gain access to the body, particularly following industrial exposure. We will discuss the *metals* and metallic ions under a separate heading, although many would perhaps fit more happily under the autogenous and exogenous headings.

Artefactual pigments

The most important of these is *formalin pigment*, a brownish-black deposit which is found in formalin-fixed tissues, particularly where there is a large amount of blood in the tissue, e.g. spleen, lung infarct, cerebral haemorrhage. It can be eradicated by pretreating the slide in alcoholic picric acid for two hours or longer before staining. Very closely related to formalin pigment is *malarial pigment*; this is also brownish-black and is similarly cleared by alcoholic picric acid. It occurs as a deposit over red cells which contain malarial parasites.

A brown-black *mercury pigment* will occur in sections prepared from tissues fixed in a mercury-containing fixative, i.e. formol sublimate. This is easily cleared from the tissue sections by treatment with iodine and sodium thiosulphate before staining.

A fine yellow dichromate deposit may be found in tissue which has been inadequately washed following fixation in any of the dichromate fixatives. The deposit can be removed by treating the section with acid alcohol for 20–30 minutes.

Fixation pigments are summarised in Table 8.1.

Table 8.1. Fixation pigments

Pigment	Appearance	Removed by
Formalin pigment	Dark brown/black granules (non-birefringent)	Alcoholic picric acid
Malarial pigment	Dark brown/black granules (birefringent)	Alcoholic picric acid
Mercury pigment	Coarse black crystals	Iodine, thiosulphate
Dichromate pigment	Fine yellow deposit	Acid alcohol

Autogenous pigments

HAEMOGLOBIN

Haemoglobin may be easily demonstrated by peroxidase methods based on benzidine. Unfortunately this chemical compound is known to be carcinogenic and is being withdrawn from the market. However, the need positively to demonstrate haemoglobin in tissue sections rarely arises. The leuco patent blue V method also relies upon the reaction of haemoglobin peroxidase.

LIPOFUSCIN

This is probably the most widely occurring natural pigment in human tissues. It is a golden-brown pigment found particularly in liver cells and cardiac muscle cells, usually more concentrated around the nucleus. Lipofuscin is found in increasing amounts with increasing age, and has been given the uninformative name of 'wear and tear' pigment. Its exact nature, mode of production and significance are unknown but it is probably a breakdown product of lipids and lipoproteins. It is attractively demonstrated by the long Ziehl–Neelsen method which stains the pigment red, and by the Sudan black method which stains it black, in some instances in paraffin sections. The method of choice is the Schmorl reaction which demonstrates lipofuscin as green-blue particles; this method, however, also demonstrates melanins and argentaffin granules, so is not selective for lipofuscin.

BILE

Histologically bile is most frequently encountered in sections of liver, and the presence of excessive amounts of bile in the liver is suggestive of intra- or extra-hepatic biliary obstruction. In H & E stained sections bile appears as golden-brown globules, beads or smooth-surfaced cylinders between hepatocytes, and no difficulty is usually encountered in identifying it for what it is. In cases of difficulty it should be remembered that bile stains a characteristic green colour with van Gieson's stain.

The time-honoured method of Gmelin is usually unnecessary; the green colour produced by the addition of alcoholic nitric acid is very transient and the whole procedure, which must be performed on the microscope stage, is messy.

MELANIN

Melanin is a normal tissue pigment and occurs in the melanocytes and melanophores of the skin. More important clinically is the fact that melanin is produced by the malignant tumour, malignant melanoma, and the ability to demonstrate small quantities of melanin within the cells of an anaplastic tumour say, for instance, in a lymph node, may have considerable clinical importance. In unstained and H & E stained sections melanins appear dark brown or black; in large concentrations it is black and is fairly distinctive. In more moderate concentrations it is usually brown and may be easily confused with haemosiderin (q.v.); in small concentrations it is easily missed and special stains are needed to detect and identify it (Fig. 8.1).

Melanin has the ability to reduce silver solutions on its own without the use of a reducing agent. Ammoniacal silver techniques are therefore used for the demonstration of melanin in tissues. In all the silver methods, melanin

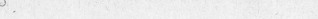

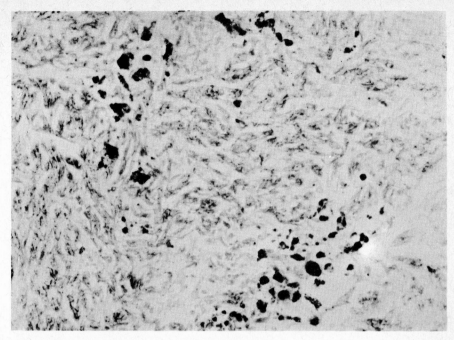

Figure 8.1 An axillary lymph node replaced by anaplastic spindle celled tumour whose nature was un-known; a small amount of brown pigment within it was thought to be haemosiderin. A Schmorl stain showed the pigment to be melanin. The patient had had a 'mole' removed from his back six months previously Magnification (× 392)

stains black; of the silver methods available we prefer the Masson–Fontana technique. The Schmorl reaction, which shows melanin dark blue by reduction of ferric ferricyanide, is also recommended (see Table 8.4).

Cells capable of producing melanin possess the enzyme tyrosinase (dopa-oxidase) which catalyses the oxidation of tyrosine to dihydroxyphenylalanine (dopa) and also the final oxidation of dopa to melanin. This enzyme can be demonstrated quite simply, but it is necessary to use either freshly fixed blocks of tissue or freshly fixed cryostat sections; it is not applicable to long-fixed tissues or paraffin-embedded tissue.

Chromaffin, argentaffin and argyrophil

There is considerable confusion over these words, the more so since they were originally coined on the basis of staining reactions and are not mutually exclusive. The words are applied to certain staining reactions of cells which, though found in many different sites in the body, share the common feature that they are responsible for the production of certain amines.

So-called *chromaffin* cells contain granules which do not stain with formalin-fixed H & E, but which have an affinity for chromates and become yellow-brown when treated by chromate solution. The chromaffin reaction may be weakly positive in formalin-fixed tissues which are post-chromed in dichromate. They are classically found in the cells of the adrenal medulla and its most common tumour, phaeochromocytoma. The chromaffin granules in this situation contain high concentrations of adrenaline, noradrenaline and their precursors. Noradrenaline can be more specifically identified in formalin-fixed frozen sections or in freeze-dried formalin vapour-fixed sections using the fluorescence technique of Eranko ; noradrenaline shows strong fluorescence. The chromaffin granules also show reducing activity when the tissue has been fixed in formalin ; therefore they have the ability to reduce silver solutions and are thus stained black by the Masson–Fontana and other silver methods. Chromate fixation destroys this ability.

Chromaffin-containing tissues which are fixed in a dichromate-containing fixative, such as Regaud's fluid, can be stained with Leishman or Giemsa stains, the chromaffin cells staining a characteristic yellow-green colour. Chromaffin cells are stained greenish-blue by Schmorl's method after chromate fixation.

Certain cells within the lining epithelium of the alimentary tract show a modified chromaffin reaction ; they only demonstrate the chromaffin reaction with potassium dichromate *after* they have previously been treated with formalin. True chromaffin tissue, however, gives the yellow-brown staining reaction with dichromate directly. In fact, the reaction is greatly impaired if there has been previous exposure to formalin. Nevertheless, these alimentary tract cells have been called *entero-chromaffin* cells on the basis of this modified chromaffin reaction. These cells are also known as *Kultchitsky* cells and are normally found at the base of intestinal glands, in the mucosa of the appendix and in parts of the gastric mucosa. They also reduce ammoniacal silver solutions directly (with the production of black metallic silver) in the dark, and are consequently more commonly known as *argentaffin* cells. The positive argentaffin reaction is also shown by the tumour of Kultchitsky cells, the carcinoid tumour, often called an argentaffinoma.

When such a silver reduction method (e.g. Masson–Fontana) is applied to a section of, say, intestine, the argentaffin cells stain black. If the reaction is carried out in the light, or if a reducing agent is added, many more cells will stain black. These cells which only reduce silver if an external reducing agent is added, are called *argyrophil* cells, and are more numerous and more widely distributed than true argentaffin cells.

The true argentaffin cells show the argentaffin reaction because they contain an amine, 5-hydroxytryptamine (serotonin) in high concentration. The argyrophil cells need the additional help of an external reducing agent because they contain much smaller quantities of the amine.

Argentaffin granules are well demonstrated by the diazo reaction.

In summary therefore :

Chromaffin cells contain granules which stain yellow-brown when fixed in dichromate solution ; this reaction is largely destroyed if the tissue is fixed in formalin previously. These granules have reducing abilities and will reduce silver solutions to form black metallic silver if previously fixed in formalin ; chromate fixation destroys this reaction. In other words, true chromaffin cells will show a positive argentaffin reaction under specific circumstances.

Argentaffin cells have the ability to reduce silver solutions directly in the dark, without the aid of an external reducing agent. Only if argentaffin cells have been fixed in formalin will they show the chromaffin reaction with dichromate, a distinction from true chromaffin cells.

Argyrophil cells also have the ability to reduce silver solutions, but need assistance in the way of an external reducing agent.

True chromaffin cells are best demonstrated by the chromaffin reaction, or by a Giemsa stain.

Argentaffin cells stain black with a silver method such as the Masson–Fontana.

Argyrophil cells are best demonstrated by a silver method which includes an external reducing agent, such as Bodian's silver proteinate method.

Metals and metallic ions

IRON (haemosiderin)

Iron is absorbed in the small intestine and transported to the bone marrow where most of it is stored (as the brown ferric iron–protein complex called haemosiderin) ready for release when required for incorporation into the haemoglobin molecule in normal erythropoiesis. When the life span of the red cells is over their cell walls are destroyed in the lymphoreticular system, usually in the spleen, and the iron is split off from the haemoglobin molecule and most recirculates to the marrow where it is again stored as haemosiderin. Stainable (ferric) iron is therefore found normally in the bone marrow, and in small quantities in the spleen. It is found in excessive amounts if abnormally large quantities of iron enter the body over a long period of time, either in the form of blood (transfusion haemosiderosis) or as intramuscular or intravenous therapeutic preparations, or if there is excessive breakdown of blood, as in haemolytic conditions, or in the disease known as haemochromatosis (Fig. 8.2) in which large amounts of dietary iron are absorbed indiscriminately by the intestinal mucosa. In all of these cases the demonstrable iron is found mainly in the lymphoreticular system, particularly in liver, spleen and lymph nodes. Iron may be found in many other sites, in fact anywhere where there has been local destruction of red cells, for example in areas of haemorrhage, infarction, longstanding congestion, and trauma. Ferric iron is satisfactorily demonstrated by Perls' Prussian blue reaction. In this reaction loosely bound iron is separated from the protein to which it is attached by dilute HCl; the ferric iron thus released reacts with dilute potassium ferrocyanide to produce ferric ferrocyanide, an insoluble blue compound. A red counterstain is usually incorporated into the method. Ferrous iron, which is of little clinical significance, can be demonstrated by Tirmann's method.

CALCIUM

Calcium appears on H & E stained sections as blue–purple material, either in shapeless irregular masses, or in thin lines if the calcium salts have been deposited on fibres, e.g. on the elastic laminae of old arteries. Calcium can be positively identified by two methods, *von Kossa's technique* (1901) and the *alizarin red S* method. Von Kossa's technique is particularly useful when applied to undecalcified bone sections and this is dealt with in detail in Chapter 7.

Alizarin red S forms a stable red lake with calcium. The method is most useful where calcium is present in small quantities, e.g. in nephrocalcinosis and other examples of heterotopic calcification; however, it is less useful than the von Kossa in bone sections.

Neither of the two stains discussed are specific for calcium, as the silver (in von Kossa's method) or alizarin red may combine with phosphates or

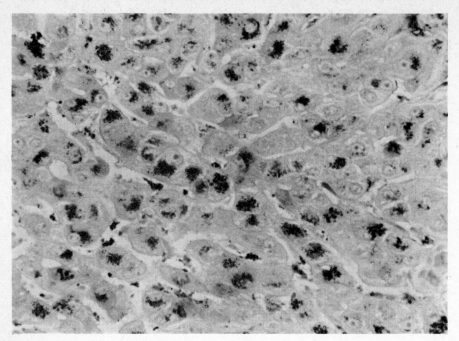

Figure 8.2 Liver from a patient with haemochromatosis. The excessive iron accumulated in the liver cells and Kupffer cells is stained dark blue by Perls' stain. Magnification (× 392)

carbonates attached to other metal ions, but from a practical point of view this rarely occurs and any material which is positive by these methods can safely be regarded as calcium.

COPPER

Copper is present in such small quantities in normal tissues that it cannot be demonstrated by histochemical methods. However, in Wilson's disease ('hepatolenticular degeneration') there is deposition of greatly excessive amounts of copper within the liver and the basal ganglia region of the brain. This copper can be demonstrated by the rubeanic acid technique, in which the rubeanic acid combines with copper to form insoluble greenish-black copper rubeanate (Fig. 8.3).

Exogenous material

CARBON

Carbon occurs as characteristic black clumps or irregular small particles and is rarely confused with other black pigments, such as melanin, on an H & E stained section. If proof is needed, carbon cannot be dissolved by concentrated sulphuric acid and is not bleached by Mayer's chlorine method. The other black pigments are soluble in the acid and are bleached by chlorine. Carbon is commonly found in the lungs and thoracic lymph nodes in city dwellers, smokers and coal miners.

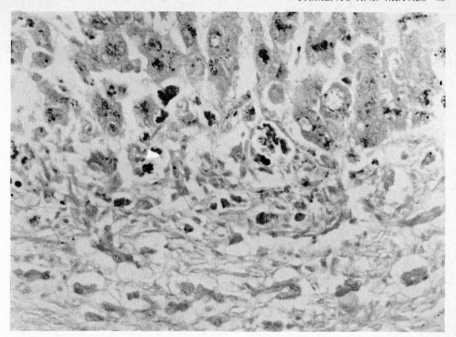

Figure 8.3 Edge of a liver lobule in cirrhosis due to Wilson's disease. The excess copper within the viable and degenerate liver cells is stained darkly by the rubeanic acid method. Magnification (× 392)

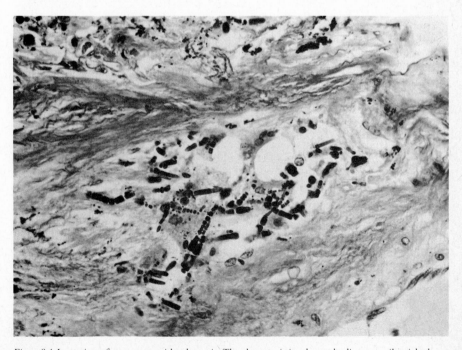

Figure 8.4 Lung tissue from a man with asbestosis. The characteristic asbestos bodies are easily picked out because they stain dark blue with Perls' stain. Magnification (× 392)

SILICA (including asbestos)

Silica is found in the lung in cases of *silicosis*. The silica particles can be detected in tissue sections because they show birefringence when viewed under crossed polaroids. A special form of silicosis is *asbestosis*; asbestos is a hydrated magnesium silicate which is present in the form of long thin

Table 8.2. Staining methods available for pigments

Staining method	Pigmentation	Pathological site	See page
Perls' Prussian blue	Ferric iron	E.g. liver	87
Tirmann and Schmeltzer	Ferrous and ferric iron	E.g. liver	87
Periodic acid Schiff	Lipofuscin	Liver, heart	19
Long Ziehl–Neelsen	Lipofuscin	Liver, heart	92
Sudan black	Lipofuscin	Liver, heart	32
Schmorl	See Table 8.4		88
Masson–Fontana	Melanin, argentaffin granules	Melanoma, carcinoid tumours	90
Diazo (alkaline)	Argentaffin granules	Carcinoid tumours	89
Dopa-oxidase	Tyrosinase, melanin	Melanomas	91
Giemsa	Chromaffin	Phaeochromocytoma	92
Toluidine blue	Chromaffin	Phaeochromocytoma	—
Rubeanic acid	Copper	Basal ganglia of brain, and liver	93

Table 8.3. Demonstration of pigments

Pigment	Recommended method	Others
Argentaffin granules	Diazo (alkaline)	Schmorl, Masson–Fontana
Chromaffin granules	(Chromaffin reaction)	Giemsa
	Dichromate fixation	
Haemoglobin	Dunn-Thompson leuco patent blue	Dunn-Thompson modified van Gieson
Haemotoidin (bile)	Van Gieson	Stein, Fouchets, Gmelin
Haemosiderin (iron)	Perls'	Quincke's
Lipofuscin	Long Ziehl–Neelsen	Schmorl, Sudan black
Melanin	Masson–Fontana	Schmorl
Copper	Rubeanic acid	–
Silica	Birefringence	Micro-incineration
Silver	Birefringence	Ammonium sulphide
Carbon	–	–
Asbestos bodies	Perls' Prussian blue	Occasionally birefringent
Lead	Haematoxylin (Mallory)	Rhodizonic acid
Haemazoin (malarial)	Birefringence	–

Note. Argentaffin cell granules and chromaffin granules may also be demonstrated by fluorescence.

crystalline needles which appear birefringent. After inhalation these asbestos needles may become coated with protein and other substances to form characteristically-shaped asbestos bodies; these may not show birefringence but the ensheathing protein usually stains blue with Perls' Prussian blue reaction, probably because of iron incorporated into the protein sheath (Fig. 8.4).

ALUMINIUM AND BERYLLIUM

These metals may rarely gain access to tissues, usually following industrial exposure. They can be demonstrated by the *naphthochrome B* method, in which metals combine with naphthochrome green B to produce a green dye lake. The metals can be distinguished the one from the other by modifying the pH of the dye solution: beryllium stains green at pH 5.0 and aluminium stains strongly at pH 7.3.

A summary of pigments and the methods available for their demonstration is given in Tables 8.2 and 8.3.

STAINING METHODS

Demonstration of iron in tissue sections

Two types of iron are found in tissue sections: ferric iron, by far the most common, is demonstrated by Perls' Prussian blue reaction, while ferrous salts are demonstrated by Tirmann's reaction. Quincke's reaction will demonstrate both ferric and ferrous iron, by converting ferric salts to ferrous, both then being demonstrated.

Prussian blue reaction (Perls, 1867)

This method will demonstrate *ferric iron*, but not ferrous iron which is demonstrated by the Tirmann's method.

SOLUTION
Perls' solution

2 per cent potassium ferrocyanide	25 ml
2 per cent hydrochloric acid	25 ml

METHOD
1. Place sections in xylol, then down to water.
2. Rinse in distilled water.
3. Transfer to Perls' solution for 15 minutes.
4. Rinse in distilled water.
5. Counterstain in 1 per cent neutral red.
6. Rinse in tap water.
7. Dehydrate, clear and mount in DPX.

RESULTS
Haemosiderin: *blue.*
Nuclei: *red.*

NOTES
1. The Perls' solution should be freshly prepared and filtered.
2. Use Analar grade reagents.
3. Other pigments will not stain.
4. Use known control slides.
5. If excessive amounts of iron are present, the staining time will need to be reduced.

Tirmann and Schmeltzer's method for ferrous and ferric iron
(Tirmann, 1898; Schmeltzer, 1933)

This method is based upon the combination of two well known chemical

G

reactions. In the Quincke (1880) reaction, ferric iron is converted to ferrous iron by the treatment with ammonium sulphide, any original ferrous iron remaining unaltered. The ferrous iron thus produced is then demonstrated by the Turnbull blue reaction in which insoluble blue ferrous ferricyanide is produced by treatment of the ferrous iron with potassium ferricyanide.

Ferrous iron alone can be demonstrated by the Turnbull blue reaction without the pretreatment with ammonium sulphide.

METHOD
1. Place sections in xylol, then down to water.
2. Rinse sections in distilled water.
3. Treat sections with dilute ammonium sulphide for 2 hours.
4. Wash well in distilled water.
5. Treat sections with a solution of equal parts of 20 per cent potassium ferricyanide and 2 per cent hydrochloric acid for 10 minutes.
6. Rinse in distilled water.
7. Counterstain in 1 per cent neutral red.
8. Wash in tap water.
9. Dehydrate, clear and mount in DPX.

RESULTS
Ferric and ferrous salts: *blue.*
Nuclei: *red.*

Schmorl's method for lipofuscins (Schmorl, 1934)
This technique is capable of demonstrating substances that are able to reduce ferricyanide (see Table 8.4 and below).

SOLUTION

1 per cent ferric chloride	37.5 ml
1 per cent potassium ferricyanide	5.0 ml
Distilled water	7.5 ml

METHOD
1. Place sections in xylol, then down to water.
2. Immerse sections in staining solution 30 seconds to 5 minutes (see note 1).
3. Rinse in tap water.
4. Place in 1 per cent acetic acid for 2 minutes.
5. Wash well in tap water.
6. Stain in 1 per cent neutral red for 2 minutes.
7. Wash in tap water.
8. Dehydrate, clear and mount in DPX.

RESULTS
Lipofuscin: *blue* to *dark blue.*
Melanin: *very dark blue.*
Argentaffin granules: *blue.*
Chromaffin granules: *greenish blue.*
Nuclei: *red.*

NOTES
1. The section should be looked at after 30 seconds to see if any staining is visible under the microscope. In the majority of cases lipofuscins and melanins will stain in 2 minutes. Other reducing substances, i.e. chromaffin granules, which are less able to reduce ferricyanide, take longer to stain and appear more greenish in colour.
2. Due to the small amounts of reducing agents present in tissue generally, background staining occurs quite rapidly and for this reason the staining time should be kept to a minimum (see note 1).
3. If ferrous iron is present in the tissue a false positive result will be obtained.
4. For the demonstration of chromaffin granules dichromate-fixed material must be used.
5. For argentaffin granules formol saline fixation must be used.
6. On some occasions difficulty may be encountered with counterstaining with 1 per cent neutral red.
7. Use known control section.
8. Stain must be freshly prepared, if the solution is green it should be discarded.
9. 1 per cent ferric nitrate may be used instead of the chloride.

Table 8.4. Staining reactions with Schmorl reaction

Pigments	Fixative	Colour	Rate
Lipofuscin	Any	Dark blue	Fast
Melanin	Any	Very dark blue	Fast
Argentaffin granules	Formol saline	Blue	Slow
Chromaffin granules	Dichromate	Greenish-blue	Slow

Alkaline diazo reaction for argentaffin cell granules

This method will demonstrate argentaffin cell granules in the small intestine and in carcinoid tumours.

SOLUTION
Incubating solution

Fast red B salt	50 mg
0.1M veronal acetate buffer pH 9.2	50 ml
or	
1 per cent aqueous fast red B salt	5 ml
Saturated lithium carbonate	2 ml

METHOD
1. Place sections in xylol, then down to water.
2. Transfer to incubating medium for 30 seconds to 1 minute.
3. Wash well in running tap water for 5–10 minutes.
4. Stain nuclei in haemalum for 3 minutes.
5. Wash well in tap water.
6. Differentiate in 1 per cent acid alcohol.
7. Wash well in tap water for 5 minutes.
8. Dehydrate, clear and mount in DPX.

RESULTS
Argentaffin cell granules: *orange* to *red*.
Nuclei: *blue*.

NOTES
1. Rapid fixation is critical, and for this reason the method often fails with necropsy material.
2. In some carcinoid tumours a weak result may be obtained; tumours of the appendix and small bowel are usually positive, bronchial 'carcinoids' are almost invariably negative.
3. Other azo dyes may be used.
4. Best results are obtained with the incubating solution at 4°C.
5. Use known control section.

Masson–Fontana method for melanin (Masson, 1928)
This method will also stain the argentaffin cells of the small intestine.

SOLUTION
Fontana silver solution

10 per cent silver nitrate	20 ml
Ammonia	
Distilled water	20 ml

To 10 per cent silver nitrate add strong ammonia drop by drop until only a faint opalescence remains. Add the distilled water and filter. Allow to stand overnight before use. If kept in the dark the solution will keep for up to one month. Never use the same staining solution more than three times.

METHOD
1. Place sections in xylol, then down to water.
2. Wash in distilled water.
3. Transfer to Fontana silver solution overnight in the dark in covered container.
4. Wash well in two changes of distilled water.
5. Fix sections in 5 per cent sodium thiosulphate for 5 minutes.
6. Wash in tap water for 5 minutes.
7. Counterstain in 1 per cent neutral red for 2 minutes.
8. Dehydrate, clear and mount in DPX.

RESULTS
Melanin: *black*.
Nuclei: *red*.

NOTES
1. With longer incubation in the silver solution argentaffin cell granules can be demonstrated.
2. Sections may be toned in gold chloride after stage 4, if required.
3. A known positive control section should be used.
4. Lipofuscin may also stain occasionally.

5. An explosive compound can develop with ammoniacal silver solution (Wallington, 1965).

Dopa-oxidase (Tyrosinase, dopa reaction; Becker, Praver and Thatcher, 1935)

This method will demonstrate tyrosinase in tissue sections. The technique given below is applied to small blocks of tissue, after which paraffin sections are cut (method 1). Laidlaw and Blackberg's (1932) modification can be applied to frozen sections and this (method 2) is ideal for cryostat material.

SOLUTION
Incubating solution

DL-3,4-dihydroxyphenylalanine (dopa)	100 mg	
0.1M phosphate buffer (pH 7.4)	100 ml	

METHOD 1
1. Fix small pieces of tissue (1–2 mm) in 10 per cent formal saline for 1 hour.
2. Wash in running tap water.
3. Place tissues in incubating solution at 37°C for 1 hour.
4. Transfer blocks to fresh incubating solution at 37°C overnight.
5. Wash tissues in running tap water for 10 minutes.
6. Fix blocks in 10 per cent formol saline overnight.
7. Dehydrate blocks through graded alcohols to absolute alcohol.
8. Clear in chloroform or toluene.
9. Embed in paraffin wax.
10. Cut sections 5 μ thick.
11. Dewax and take down to water.
12. Counterstain in Mayer's carmalum.
13. Wash in tap water.
14. Dehydrate through graded alcohols to xylene, mount in DPX.

RESULTS
Tyrosinase: *dark brown granules.*
Nuclei: *red.*

METHOD 2
This technique is applied to formalin-fixed frozen sections; post-fixed cryostat sections are ideal.
1. Wash sections in distilled water.
2. Transfer sections to incubating solution at 37°C for 45 minutes.
3. Immerse sections in fresh incubating solution at 37°C for 2–3 hours (see note).
4. Wash in running tap water for 5 minutes.
5. Counterstain in Mayer's carmalum if required.
6. Dehydrate through graded alcohols to xylene, mount in DPX.

RESULTS
Tyrosinase activity: *brownish black.*
Nuclei: *red.*

NOTE

In method 2 the time required in the incubating solution should be judged by looking at the section microscopically at 30-minute intervals.

Long Ziehl–Neelsen for Lipofuscin

SOLUTION

Carbol fuchsin	Basic fuchsin	1 g
	Phenol	0.5 g
	Absolute alcohol	10 ml
	Distilled water	100 ml

METHOD
1. Place sections in xylol, then down to water.
2. Place sections in carbol fuchsin at 60°C for 3 hours.
3. Wash well in tap water.
4. Differentiate in 1 per cent acid alcohol till RBCs are light pink.
5. Wash well in tap water.
6. Counterstain lightly in Mayer's haemalum.
7. Wash in tap water.
8. Dehydrate, clear and mount in DPX.

RESULTS
Lipofuscin: *red*.
Nuclei: *blue*.

NOTE

Sections may be left in the stain for a longer period if required.

Giemsa method for chromaffin cell granules

This is a satisfactory method of demonstrating chromaffin granules following dichromate fixation.

SOLUTION
Dilute Giemsa stain

| Standard Giemsa stain | 2 ml |
| Buffered distilled water pH 6.8 | 48 ml |

METHOD
1. Place sections in xylol, then down to water.
2. Rinse in distilled water.
3. Stain in dilute Giemsa stain overnight.
4. Rinse in distilled water.
5. Wash in 0.5 per cent acetic acid till section is pink, 2 minutes.
6. Wash in tap water.
7. Dehydrate rapidly, clear and mount.

RESULTS
Chromaffin cell granules: *greenish yellow*.
Nuclei: *blue*.

NOTES
1. Dehydration must be rapid.
2. The concentration of the stain is not critical.

Rubeanic acid method for copper (Okamoto and Utamura, 1938; Uzman, 1956; Howell, 1959)

SOLUTION

Rubeanic acid staining solution

0.1 per cent rubeanic acid in absolute alcohol	2.5 ml
10 per cent sodium acetate	50 ml

METHOD
1. Place sections in xylol, then down to water.
2. Stain section in rubeanic acid staining solution at 37°C overnight.
3. Place sections in 70 per cent alcohol for 15 minutes.
4. Transfer sections to absolute alcohol for 6 hours.
5. Rinse in fresh absolute alcohol.
6. Clear in xylol and mount in DPX.

RESULT
Copper: *greenish black granules.*

NOTES
1. Sections tend to lift, so always stain spare sections.
2. Normal physiological quantities of copper are not demonstrated (see text).
3. Counterstain with alcoholic eosin if required.

Leuco-dye method for haemoglobin peroxidase (Dunn-Thompson, 1946; Lison, 1938)

The enzyme is reasonably resistant to formalin fixation; times exceeding 48 hours are not recommended.

SOLUTIONS
Stock solution

Patent blue	1 g
Distilled water	100 ml
Powdered zinc	10 g
Glacial acetic acid	2 ml

Add the reagents in the order given. Boil the solution until it becomes colourless. Cool and filter immediately before use.

Leuco blue incubating solution

Stock solution	10 ml
Glacial acetic acid	2 ml
3 per cent hydrogen peroxide	1 ml

METHOD
1. Place sections in xylol, then down to water.
2. Immerse sections in leuco blue solution for 5 minutes.
3. Rinse in tap water.
4. Counterstain in 1 per cent neutral red for 1 minute.
5. Rinse in tap water.
6. Dehydrate through graded alcohols to xylene and mount in DPX.

RESULTS
Haemoglobin: *dark blue.*
Other oxidase granules: *dark blue.*
Nuclei: *red.*

REFERENCES

BECKER, S. W., PRAVER, L. L. & THATCHER, H. (1935). An improved (paraffin section) method for the dopa reaction. *Arch. Derm. Syph.*, **31**, 190.

HOWELL, J. S. (1959). Histochemical demonstration of copper in copper fed rats and in the hepatolenticular degeneration. *J. Path. Bact.*, **77**, 423.

KOSSA, J. VON (1901). Ueber die im organismus Kunstlich eizeugberen verkalkungen. *Beitr. path. Anat.*, **29**, Suppl. 4, 163.

LAIDLAW, G. F. & BLACKBERG, S. N. (1932). Melanoma studies; dopa reaction in normal histology. *Amer. J. Path.*, **8**, 491.

MASSON, P. (1928). Carcinoids and nerve hyperplasia of appendicular mucosa. *Amer. J. Path.*, **4**, 181.

OKAMOTO, K. & UTAMURA, M. (1938). Biologische untersuchungen des kupfers; uber die histochemische kupfernachweis methode. *Trans. Soc. Path. Japan*, **20**, 573.

PERLS, M. (1867). Nachweis von eisenoxyd in gewissen pigmenten. *Virchows Arch. path. Anat.*, **39**, 42.

QUINCKE, H. (1880). Zur Pathologie des Blutes. *Dt. Arch. klin. Med.*, **25**, 567.

SCHMELTZER, W. (1933). Der mikrochemische nachweis von eisen in Gewebselementen mittels Rhoden-wasserswtoffsaure und die konservierung der reaktion in paraffinol. *Z. wiss. Mikr.*, **50**, 99.

SCHMORL, G. (1934). *Die pathologisch-histologischen untersuchungs methoden*, 16th edition, ed. Geipel, P. Berlin: Vogel.

TIRMANN, J. (1898). Ueber den Uebergang des eisens in die milch. *Gorbersdorfer veroffentlichungen*, **2**, 101.

UZMAN, L. L. (1956). Histochemical localization of copper with rubeanic acid. *Lab. Invest.*, **5**, 299.

WALLINGTON, E. A. (1965). The explosive properties of ammoniacal silver solutions. *J. med. Lab. Technol.*, **22**, 220.

FURTHER READING

BANCROFT, J. D. (1975). *An Introduction to Histochemical Technique*, 2nd edition. London: Butterworths (in Press).

CULLING, C. F. A. (1963). *Handbook of Histopathological Techniques*, 2nd edition. London: Butterworths.

DISBREY, B. D. & RACK, J. H. (1970). *Histological Laboratory Methods*. Edinburgh & London: Livingstone.

DRURY, R. A. B. & WALLINGTON, E. A. (1967). *Carleton's Histological Technique*, 4th edition. Oxford University Press.

PEARSE, A. G. E. (1972). *Histochemistry, Theoretical and Applied*, Vol. 2, pp. 1050–1101. Edinburgh & London: Churchill Livingstone.

CHAPTER 9

Microorganisms

The most commonly used stain to demonstrate bacteria in tissue sections is Gram's stain. Using this method bacteria can be classified into two main groups: Gram-positive bacteria in which the organisms stain blue-black, and Gram-negative bacteria which are stained red (Table 9.1).

Certain bacteria are not satisfactorily demonstrated by the Gram stain; most important of these are the mycobacterial organisms which, because of their lipid capsule, are very resistant to staining. The *Ziehl–Neelsen* stain was developed to demonstrate tubercle bacilli, and remains the most commonly used method of demonstrating mycobacterial organisms in use (Ziehl, 1882;

Table 9.1. Classification of bacteria by Gram stain

Gram-positive bacteria		Gram-negative bacteria	
Cocci	*Bacilli*	*Cocci*	*Bacilli*
Staphylococci	Bacillus	Neisseriae	Escherischia
e.g. *S. aureus*	e.g. *B. anthracis*	e.g. *N. gonorrhoeae*	e.g. *E. coli*
Streptococci	Clostridia		Shigellae
e.g. *S. pyogenes*	e.g. *C. welchii*		e.g. *S. sonnei*
	Corynebacteria		Salmonellae
	e.g. *C. diphtheriae*		e.g. *S. typhi*
			Proteus
			e.g. *P. vulgaris*
			Haemophilus
			e.g. *H. influenzae*
			Bordetella
			e.g. *B. pertussis*
			Pseudomonas
			e.g. *Ps. aeruginosa*
			Klebsiella
			e.g. *K. pneumoniae*

Neelsen, 1883). Examining a histological section for very small numbers of minute red-stained organisms is an irritating and time-consuming chore; however, a simple and quick fluorescent method is becoming increasingly used in routine laboratories. It is based on the work of Matthaei (1950) and modified by Kuper and May (1960). The tubercle bacilli shine brightly yellow against a dark background and are much more readily picked up than on a ZN stained section.

Spirochaetes are also difficult to demonstrate in tissue sections; the method of choice is the Warthin and Starry (1920) technique which has replaced the old Levaditi method.

Fungi

Most fungi can be seen on haematoxylin and eosin stained sections, although Nocardia and Candida are very difficult to detect. The Aspergillus species are lightly stained by haematoxylin, but can be demonstrated with much more ease by special stains. The best of these for Aspergillus are the *Grocott–Gomori methenamine silver* stain (Grocott, 1953) and *Gridley's modified PAS reaction* (Gridley, 1953) and these are widely acceptable for the demonstration of all fungi. The unmodified PAS reaction is used particularly to demonstrate *Candida albicans* and the many dermatophytic fungi; these organisms are PAS positive because of the high carbohydrate content of their cell walls.

Cryptococci can be demonstrated in two ways. The organism itself is stained black by the *Grocott–Gomori method* whilst the thick capsule around the yeast cells appears as a non-staining 'halo'. An alternative, but less satisfactory, method is to stain the mucoid capsule using Southgate's mucicarmine.

COMMON FUNGI

Aspergillus fumigatus is most commonly seen in man as a pathogen when it infects old lung cavities, such as those left by old tuberculous infection, and as a diffuse lung infection (sometimes becoming systematised via the blood stream) in patients who have a suppressed immune response for some reason. The organism is seen as a mycelium of broad, branching septate hyphae. Very occasionally the characteristic fruiting body, the conidiophore, is seen in tissue sections (Fig. 9.1b); they are most likely to be seen where the organism is in contact with the air, for example when the fungus is in a bronchus. Aspergillus has the ability to infiltrate through vessel walls, even arteries (Fig. 9.1a), and so can sometimes be seen to be causing a very localised 'arteritis', and the hyphae can often be seen within thrombotic material.

Candida albicans can infect the mouth and pharynx ('thrush'), the oesophagus, the vagina (vaginal moniliasis), the skin, finger and toe-nails, and the perianal region. In babies the latter gives rise to a very severe form of 'nappy rash'. Infection by *Candida albicans* can become systematised, giving rise to scattered Candida abscesses throughout the body, particularly the kidney. This occurs mostly in immunosuppressed patients, in patients on long term intravenous therapy, and in mainline heroin addicts. In bloodstream infection the organisms often settle on the heart valves producing the florid vegetations of a fungal endocarditis.

The organism exists in two forms, as a matted mycelium of 'pseudohyphae', and as discrete round or ovoid yeast-like bodies. Often the early pseudohyphae can be seen apparently 'budding off' from yeast forms. In a well-established infection, particularly on an epithelial surface, the pseudohyphae are the most numerous, although yeast forms can always be found. In earlier lesions, particularly within solid internal organs, as in a small abscess arising from a blood-borne infection, the yeast forms predominate but some show early pseudohypha formation.

Cryptococcus neoformans gives rise to a very severe meningitis, often resistant to treatment. The portal of entry is the lung where the yeasts give rise to an area of whitish consolidation, often small and usually at the periphery of the lung; in lung lesions the alveoli are often packed with cryptococci. In the meningitis the organisms are found in large numbers in the subarachnoid space and sometimes within the brain itself, occasionally forming a slimy

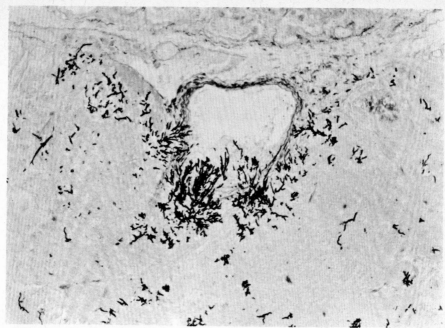

Figure 9.1 (a) Lung tissue stained by the Grocott–Gomori methenamine silver stain to demonstrate the black-staining hyphae of *Aspergillus fumigatus*. Note that the fungus is penetrating the wall of a vessel. From a 23-year-old woman who died of systematised aspergillosis three months after a renal transplant. Magnification (× 101)

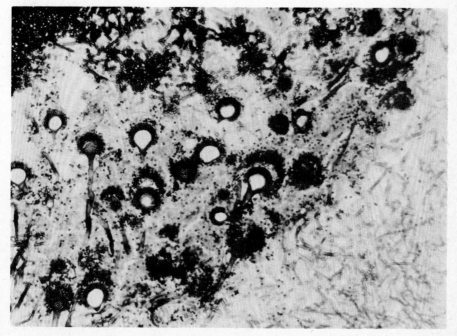

(b) Bronchial contents from the same patient showing the conidiophores of *Aspergillus fumigatus*, stained by the Grocott–Gomori methenamine silver stain. Magnification (× 252)

mucoid abscess. In both the lung and the meninges the cellular response to the yeasts is variable: sometimes polymorphonuclear, sometimes histiocytic, and very frequently very little cellular response at all.

Actinomyces israelii is probably more truly a form of bacterium rather than a true fungus, but taxonomists are still in dispute over the matter. Infection occurs most commonly in the glands in the neck and occasionally in the appendix. The H & E appearance of the colonies ('sulphur granules') and the numerous small abscesses they produce are well known; the Gram stain is a useful adjunct sometimes. Actinomyces are commonly found in the mouth, and are frequently seen as a non-pathogenic commensal in histological sections of tonsils, deep in the crypts, as an incidental finding.

A WORD OF CAUTION

Certain fungi grow very happily in many of the reagents and stains which are applied to histological sections. Inevitably, despite all precautions, fungal elements are deposited on sections and are not removed during subsequent processing. Similar problems are occasionally encountered in the summer months when pollen grains floating in the air may be deposited on sections; some types of pollen look like bizarre yeasts. In both cases the extraneous elements are 'above' rather than 'in' the sections, and of course are not associated with any cellular response.

Viruses and rickettsiae

Rickettsiae in tissues can be demonstrated by Macchiavello's (basic fuchsin–methylene blue) technique: rickettsiae and some viral inclusions (e.g. Negri bodies) stain red against a blue background. Viruses are too small to be seen on light microscopy, but under certain circumstances they aggregate to produce visible viral 'inclusion bodies' in the nucleus or cytoplasm of infected cells. A number of stains can be used to demonstrate viral inclusions, of which Lendrum's phloxine tartrazine and Mann's methyl blue–eosin are the most well known. The latter method has been mainly used to demonstrate the intracytoplasmic inclusion bodies (Negri bodies) in the neurones of the brain in cases of rabies; in our hands it has rarely been successful, although our experience is limited. The phloxine tartrazine method demonstrates certain viral inclusions very well (e.g. measles viral inclusions), but requires very careful differentiation under microscopic control (Fig. 9.2). It is, therefore, of little value as a 'search' stain; in our opinion the best search stain for viral inclusions is a well-performed haematoxylin and eosin. Some viral inclusions can be seen very easily on H & E, particularly those of cytomegalovirus and the virus of molluscum contagiosum; others require a more careful search, particularly the intranuclear inclusions in herpes infections. Here the pathologist's experience in selecting the most likely areas and cells for detailed search will increase the chances of detection.

The virus inclusion bodies can often be seen much more easily in 1 μ araldite-embedded toluidine blue-stained sections, although sampling problems arise because for technical reasons only small blocks of tissue can be examined. The araldite-embedded blocks can be trimmed down on a pyramitome and fruitful areas can be prepared for electron microscopy. Under the electron microscope the individual virus particles may be identified and the inclusion bodies are seen easily.

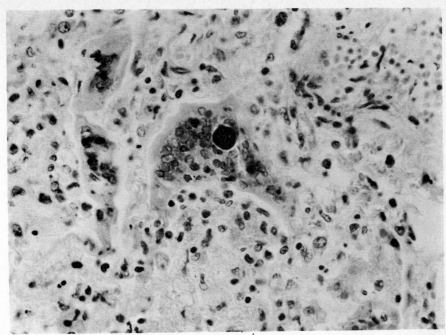

Figure 9.2 A section of lung from a child with fatal measles pneumonia. A giant cell contains large and small dark-staining viral inclusions. Lendrum's phloxine–tartrazine method. Magnification (× 392)

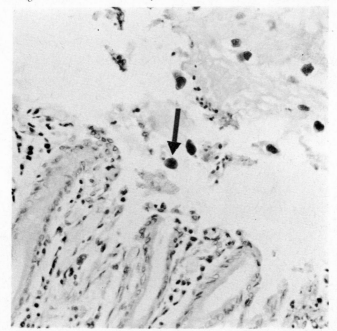

Figure 9.3 A photograph taken from the edge of a colonic ulcer, showing colonic mucosa and overlying mucus. The mucus contains numerous amoebae (arrowed), stained darkly purple by the PAS reaction. Many other amoebae were found in the depths of the ulcer. From a case of amoebic colitis. Magnification (× 252)

Protozoons and others

Amoebae are lightly stained by H & E, but are much easier to see in a PAS-stained section (Fig. 9.3). In amoebic colitis they should be particularly sought in the slough in the ulcers and in the overlying mucus in more normal areas.

Pneumocystis carinii is an important cause of severe lung infection, particularly in immunosuppressed patients such as renal transplant recipients. The histological picture in an H & E stained section of the lung is characteristic, the alveolar spaces being filled with a pale, eosinophilic, granular, rather foamy material. Careful examination under oil immersion will reveal minute dot-like, slightly haematoxyphilic organisms; they are more clearly seen in methacrylate-embedded $1\,\mu$ sections and, in normal paraffin-embedded $5\,\mu$ sections, can be picked out more clearly by the Giemsa stain. An easier way of diagnosing Pneumocystis pneumonia, however, is by using the Grocott–Gomori methenamine silver stain: the cyst walls of the encysted form of the organism are stained black. They appear as smooth, round or oval, evenly-stained bodies resembling large black erythrocytes, and are absolutely characteristic of *Pneumocystis carinii* (see Fig. 9.4).

Leishmania can be seen adequately on a good H & E stained section, but the Giemsa stain may be useful in difficult cases. The Giemsa stain can also be used to demonstrate Histoplasma, Toxoplasma and Pneumocystis organisms.

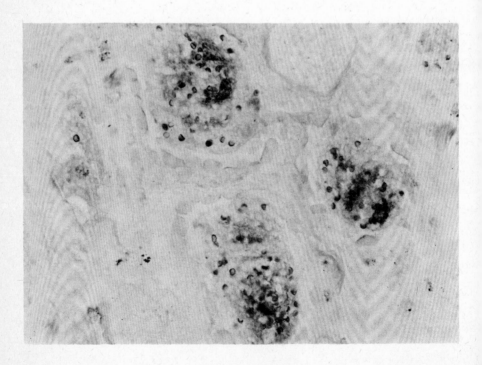

Figure 9.4 Lung tissue from a renal transplant recipient who died with extensive lung consolidation. The alveolar spaces are filled with foamy exudate in which encysted forms of *Pneumocystis carinii* can be seen, stained black by the Grocott–Gomori methenamine silver stain. Magnification (× 252)

A summary of stains for microorganisms is given in Table 9.2.

Table 9.2. Useful stains for microorganisms

Staining method	Demonstrate	Page
Gram	Gram positive and negative bacteria	101, 102
Ziehl–Neelsen	Acid-fast bacilli	103
Fluorescence	Acid-fast bacilli	103
Phloxine–tartrazine	Viral inclusion bodies	107
Gridley	Fungi	105
Grocott–Gomori's methenamine silver	Fungi, including cryptococci Pneumocystis	106
PAS	Fungi, amoebae	19
Southgate mucicarmine	Cryptococci	21
Giemsa	Protozoa (Histoplasma, Leishmania and Toxoplasma, Pneumocystis)	92
Warthin and Starry	Spirochaetes	104

STAINING METHODS FOR BACTERIA

Gram stain (Gram, 1884)

This long-established technique is not an easy one to perform as its success depends upon the decolourising stage which can only be accurately judged by experience. The technique divides the bacteria into two groups, Gram-positive and Gram-negative. There are many variations of the original method of Gram, the one given below having worked well in our hands. The Gram stain is a regressive one as both types will stain. The Gram-positive bacteria will retain the dye, whilst the Gram-negative bacteria will be decolourised by the acetone mixture and stained by the neutral red. It can be seen that over- or under-differentiation will cause complete failure of the method. For inexperienced workers the modifications of Twort (1924) or Humberstone (1963) are probably easier to use.

SOLUTIONS

Crystal violet (Lillie)

Crystal violet	2 g
95 per cent alcohol	20 ml
Ammonium oxalate	1 g
Distilled water	80 ml

Gram's iodine (will deteriorate)

Iodine crystals	1 g
Potassium iodide	2 g
Distilled water	300 ml

Iodine acetone solution

Lugol's iodine	2 ml
Acetone	98 ml

METHOD (modified)
1. Place sections in xylol, then down to water.
2. Stain in crystal violet for 45 seconds.
3. Rinse in tap water.
4. Place in Gram's iodine for 1 minute.
5. Differentiate in iodine acetone until no more colour comes from the section, 5 seconds.
6. Wash in tap water for 30 seconds.
7. Stain in 1 per cent neutral red for 1 minute.
8. Rapidly rinse in tap water.
9. Dehydrate, clear and mount.

RESULTS
Gram-positive organisms: *blue-black.*
Gram-negative organisms: *red.*
Cell nuclei: *red.*

NOTES
1. The crystal violet solution should be filtered before use.
2. Differentiation is difficult, the iodine acetone solution should be applied evenly over the section or uneven staining will be seen.
3. The iodine added to the acetone slows the rate of differentiation, and with considerable practice the iodine may be omitted.
4. Known positive controls should always be used.

Gram-Twort method (Gram, 1884; Twort, 1924; Ollet, 1947, 1951)

SOLUTIONS
Twort's stain (modified)

0.2 per cent absolute alcoholic neutral red	9 ml
0.2 per cent absolute alcoholic fast green FCF	1 ml
Distilled water	30 ml
Mix just before use.	

METHOD
1. Place sections in xylol, then down to water.
2. Stain in crystal violet solution (see previous method) for 3 minutes.
3. Rinse in running tap water.
4. Treat with Gram's iodine (see previous method) for 3 minutes.
5. Rinse in tap water.
6. Decolourise in 2 per cent acetic acid in absolute alcohol until no more colour comes away. (The section is now a dirty brown colour).
7. Rinse rapidly in distilled water.
8. Counterstain in modified Twort's stain for 5 minutes.
9. Differentiate in 2 per cent acetic acid in absolute alcohol until no more stain comes from the section, 2 seconds.
10. Clear in xylol and mount in DPX.

RESULTS
Gram-positive organisms: *blue-black*.
Gram-negative organisms: *pink*.
Nuclei: *red*.
Background: *green*.
Red blood cells: *green*.
Elastic fibres: *black*.

Carbol fuchsin method for acid-fast bacilli (Ziehl–Neelsen)
This is the traditional method for acid-fast bacilli, still used in many laboratories, but it is being replaced in busy departments by a fluorescent method. The bacillus is contained in a lipid envelope; this makes staining difficult, but paradoxically is the basis of the ZN technique.

Carbol fuchsin is forced into the mycobacteria by heat, or by the use of a wetting agent. The section is then subjected to dilute acid which removes the red stain from the background; a suitable contrast is produced by staining the background blue.

Method (modified)
1. Place sections in xylene, then down to water.
2. Stain sections in carbol fuchsin and heat to steaming (by intermittent flaming) for 15 minutes.
3. Rinse in distilled water.
4. Differentiate in 1 per cent acid alcohol for 10 minutes.
5. Wash in 25 per cent sulphuric acid in distilled water.
6. Place in 25 per cent sulphuric acid for 3 minutes.
7. Wash in tap water for 3 minutes.
8. Counterstain in acidified methylene blue for 1 minute.
9. Rinse in tap water.
10. Dehydrate and continue to differentiate in alcohols till section is pale blue; clear and mount.

RESULTS
Acid-fast bacilli: *red*.
Background: *blue*.

NOTES
1. Control sections should be used.
2. Counterstain should be pale.
3. Flaming the section can be avoided by placing the section in carbol fuchsin for 30 minutes at 60°C.
4. Red blood cells also retain the red stain after treatment with acid.

Fluorescent method for acid-fast bacilli (Kuper and May, 1960)
This method is proving very popular as the screening time is reduced considerably from that of the ZN. The method employs the same principle as the Ziehl–Neelsen. In this instance two fluorochromes are forced into the bacillus with heat. Once stained they are resistant to decolourisation.

H

SOLUTION

Auramine O	1.5 g
Rhodamine B	0.75 g
Glycerol	75 ml
Phenol crystals (liquified at 50°C)	10 ml
Distilled water	50 ml

METHOD
1. Place sections in xylol (see note 1), then down to water.
2. Stain in auramine rhodamine solution at 60°C for 10 minutes.
3. Wash in tap water.
4. Differentiate in acid alcohol for 2 minutes.
5. Wash in tap water.
6. Place in 0.5 per cent potassium permanganate for 2 minutes.
7. Brief rinse in tap water.
8. Blot dry.
9. Rinse very rapidly in 80 per cent alcohol.
10. Blot.
11. Place in absolute alcohol.
12. Place in xylol.
13. Mount in fluoromount or DPX (see note 2).

RESULTS
Acid-fast bacilli: *bright yellow fluorescence.*
Background: *unstained* (see note 2).

NOTES
1. The removal of the paraffin wax with 1 part groundnut oil and 2 parts xylene will increase the fluorescence of the acid-fast bacilli.
2. A fluorescence-free mountant is better than DPX, but neither will prevent background fluorescence developing after the second day.

Warthin–Starry method for spirochaetes (Warthin and Starry, 1920)
   This is probably the best method available for spirochaetes. The major advantage of this technique is that it may be applied to paraffin-embedded sections; the standard Levaditi method requires treatment in silver before embedding.

SOLUTIONS
Buffer solution

Sodium acetate	1.64 g
Acetic acid	2.5 ml
Distilled water	200.0 ml

Silver solution

Silver nitrate	0.5 g
Buffer solution	50.0 ml

Developer solution

Solution 1:	Hydroquinone	300 mg ⎫	
	Buffer solution	10 ml ⎬	use 1 ml
	5 per cent scotch glue	15 ml ⎭	

Dissolve the hydroquinone in the buffer solution. From this take 1 ml, add to warmed scotch glue and store in a 37°C incubator.

Solution 2:	2 per cent silver nitrate	3 ml
	stored in a 60°C incubator.	

Mix the two solutions immediately before use.

METHOD
1. Place sections in xylol, then down to water.
2. Wash well in buffer solution.
3. Stain sections in silver solution for 1 hour at 60°C.
4. Develop sections in developer for 3 minutes at 60°C.
5. Rinse sections in tap water at 60°C.
6. Rinse sections in buffer solution.
7. Dehydrate, clear and mount.

RESULTS
Spirochaetes: *black*.
Background: *yellow-brown*.

NOTES
   Development is the critical part of the technique. A balance has to be struck between underdevelopment giving pale, thin spirochaetes on a clear background, and overdevelopment giving thick, black spirochaetes but on a dark background.

STAINING METHODS FOR FUNGI
   Although most fungi can be seen with a well-differentiated haematoxylin and eosin stain, and the majority will stain with the PAS reaction because of the carbohydrate content of the fungi, many different special stains may be used to identify the fungi. These are listed in Table 9.2.

Gridley method for fungi
   The majority of fungi are PAS positive. The Gridley method is a modification of the PAS reaction. It stains fungi selectively and is recommended rather than the standard periodic acid Schiff technique.

SOLUTIONS

Aldehyde fuchsin solution

Basic fuchsin	1 g
70 per cent alcohol	200 ml
Concentrated hydrochloric acid	2 ml
Paraldehyde	2 ml

Dissolve the fuchsin in the alcohol, then add the acid and paraldehyde. Leave at room temperature for 3 days until the solution turns deep purple, it is then ready for use. Store at 4°C and filter before use. The solution will normally keep for 3 months.

Sulphurous acid rinse

10 per cent potassium metabisulphite	7.5 ml
0.1N hydrochloric acid	7.5 ml
Distilled water	135 ml

This solution should be prepared on day of use.

METHOD
1. Place sections in xylol, then down to water.
2. Place section in 4 per cent chromic acid for 1 hour.
3. Wash in running water.
4. Place in Schiff reagent (see p. 19) for 15 minutes.
5. Rinse in sulphurous acid rinse, 3 changes of 2 minutes each.
6. Wash in running tap water for 15 minutes.
7. Stain in aldehyde fuchsin solution for 30 minutes.
8. Remove excess stain with 95 per cent alcohol.
9. Rinse in running tap water for 5 minutes.
10. Rinse in 50 per cent alcohol.
11. Stain in saturated tartrazine in cellosolve for 45 seconds.
12. Dehydrate, clear and mount.

RESULTS
Conidia: *deep red.*
Hyphae: *blue.*
Background: *yellow.*
Mucin/elastic tissue: *blue.*

NOTES
Any suitable counterstain may be used at stage 11. A good alternative to the one given is 0.25 per cent metanil yellow in 0.25 per cent acetic acid.

Grocott's method for fungi (Grocott, 1955)

This modification of Gomori's methenamine silver demonstrates fungi well. The method relies upon the reduction of the silver by aldehydes after oxidation with chromic acid.

SOLUTIONS
Methenamine silver stock solutions
Solution 1:

5 per cent sodium tetraborate in distilled water

Solution 2:

5 per cent silver nitrate in distilled water	5 ml
3 per cent methenamine (hexamine) in distilled water	100 ml

Add the methenamine solution to the silver nitrate solution. A white precipitate will form, but will clear on shaking. Both solutions 1 and 2 keep well at 4°C.

Incubating solution

Borax solution (solution 1)	5 ml
Distilled water	25 ml
Methenamine silver (solution 2)	25 ml

Light green solution

Light green	100 mg
Acetic acid	0.1 ml
Distilled water	200 ml

METHOD
1. Place sections in xylol, then down to water.
2. Oxidise in 5 per cent chromic acid for 1 hour.
3. Wash in running tap water.
4. Rinse in 1 per cent sodium bisulphite.
5. Wash in tap water for 3 minutes.
6. Rinse well in different changes of distilled water.
7. Place in silver solution for 1 hour at 60°C.
8. Wash well in distilled water.
9. Repeat wash many times.
10. Tone section in 0.1 per cent gold chloride for 4 minutes.
11. Place section in 3 per cent sodium thiosulphate for 5 minutes.
12. Wash well in tap water.
13. Lightly counterstain in light green solution for 20 seconds.
14. Wash in tap water.
15. Dehydrate, clear and mount.

RESULTS
Fungi: *black*.
Blackground: *pale green*.

NOTES
1. The sodium bisulphite removes the excess chromic acid.
2. Fibrin strands will stain but are thinner than fungi and should not cause confusion.

STAINING METHODS FOR VIRAL INCLUSIONS
Phloxine tartrazine stain (Lendrum, 1947)
   This stain is able to demonstrate many structures depending upon the

degree of differentiation. Tartrazine in cellosolve acts as both differentiator and counterstain.

SOLUTIONS

Phloxine

Phloxine	0.5 g
Calcium chloride	0.5 g
Distilled water	100 ml

Tartrazine

Saturated solution of tartrazine in
2-ethoxyethanol (cellosolve)

METHOD
1. Place sections in xylol, then down to water.
2. Stain nuclei in haematoxylin for 10 minutes.
3. Differentiate lightly in acid alcohol.
4. Wash in running tap water.
5. Stain in phloxine solution for 30 minutes.
6. Rinse in tap water.
7. Blot, then stain in tartrazine solution (see note 2).
8. Rinse in 95 per cent alcohol.
9. Dehydrate in alcohol and clear in xylol and mount in DPX.

RESULTS
Certain inclusion bodies: *bright red.*
RBC: *red.*
Paneth cell granules: *red.*
Nuclei: *blue.*
Other structures: *yellow.*

NOTES
1. The success of this method for inclusion bodies is dependent upon the differentiation with tartrazine.
2. Phloxine is removed from muscle first and inclusion bodies last, so microscopical control of stage 7 is important. Differentiation in the tartrazine is continued until the inclusion bodies are clearly seen as bright red against a yellow background. This will probably take 5 minutes or longer.

Macchiavello's technique modified (Culling, 1974)

METHOD
1. Place sections in xylol, then down to water.
2. Stain in 0.25 per cent basic fuchsin for 30 minutes.
3. Differentiate rapidly in 0.5 per cent citric acid for about 3 seconds.
4. Wash in tap water.
5. Counterstain in 1 per cent aqueous methylene blue for 15–30 seconds.
6. Wash in water.
7. Dehydrate, clear and mount in DPX.

RESULTS
Rickettsiae: *red*.
Certain viral inclusions: *red*.
Background: *blue*.

REFERENCES

CULLING, C. F. A. (1974). *Handbook of Histopathological and Histochemical Techniques*, 3rd edition. London: Butterworths.

GRAM, C. (1884). Ueber die isolirte Farbung der schizomyceten in schnitt und Trockenpaparaten. *Fortschr. med.*, **2**, 185.

GRIDLEY, M. F. (1953). A stain for fungi in tissue sections. *Amer. J. clin. Path.*, **23**, 303.

GROCOTT, R. G. (1955). A stain for fungi in tissue sections and smears. *Amer. J. clin. Path.*, **25**, 975.

HUMBERSTONE, F. D. (1963). A Gram type stain for the simultaneous demonstration of Gram positive and negative micro-organisms in paraffin sections. *J. med. Lab. Technol.*, **20**, 153.

KUPER, S. W. A. & MAY, J. R. (1960). Detection of acid fast organisms in tissue sections by fluorescence microscopy. *J. Path. Bact.*, **79**, 5.

LENDRUM, A. C. (1947). The phloxine-tartrazine method as a general histological stain and for the demonstration of inclusion bodies. *J. Path. Bact.*, **59**, 399.

MATTHAEI, E. (1950). Simplified fluorescence microscopy of tubercle bacilli. *J. gen. Microbiol.*, **4**, 393.

NEELSEN, F. (1883). Ein Casuistischer Beitrag zur Lehre von der Tuberkulose. *Zbl. med. Wiss.*, **21**, 497.

OLLETT, W. S. (1947). A method for staining both Gram-positive and Gram-negative bacteria in sections. *J. Path. Bact.*, **59**, 357.

OLLETT, W. S. (1951). Further observations on the Gram–Twort stain. *J. Path. Bact.*, **63**, 166.

TWORT, F. W. (1924). An improved neutral red light green double stain, for staining animal parasites, micro-organisms and tissues. *J. State Med.*, **32**, 351.

WARTHIN, A. S. & STARRY, A. C. (1920). A more rapid and improved method of demonstrating spirochetes in tissues. *Amer. J. Syph.*, **4**, 97.

ZIEHL, F. (1882). Zur Farbung des Tuberkelbacillus. *Dtsch. med. Wschr.*, **8**, 451.

FURTHER READING

ANTHONY, P. P. (1973). *A Guide to the Histological Identification of Fungi in Tissues. J. clin. Path.*, **26**, 828.

DISBREY, B. D. & RACK, J. H. (1970). *Histological Laboratory Methods.* Edinburgh & London: Livingstone.

DRURY, R. A. E. & WALLINGTON, E. A. (1967). *Carleton's Histological Technique*, 4th edition. Oxford University Press.

SYMMERS, W. St. C. (1960). Histological examination in the diagnosis of deep-seated fungal infections. In *Recent Advances in Clinical Pathology*, series III, ed. Dyke, S. C. London: Churchill.

CHAPTER 10

Renal Biopsies

The development of a simple, safe technique for percutaneous needle biopsy of the kidney has resulted in an enormous increase in our knowledge of the classification, diagnosis and management of renal disease. No longer has the likely renal lesion to be inferred from the symptoms, physical signs and results of laboratory investigation of blood and urine; now the lesion in the kidney can be seen, its severity assessed and, if the renal biopsy is repeated at some later date, its rate of progress or the effects of treatment can be noted. In this step forward the histopathologist has so far played a leading part and continues to do so as he adds more techniques to his repertoire.

The earliest renal biopsy specimens were processed in the normal way: fixed in formalin, embedded in paraffin wax, cut at 5μ, and stained with haematoxylin and eosin. One of the first big improvements in investigation was the preparation of sections cut on a normal microtome at 3μ from paraffin-embedded material. The thinner section enabled a much clearer view of the important glomerular features to be obtained, and changes such as marginal increase in glomerular basement membrane thickness and slight hypercellularity of the glomerular tuft were easily noticed, whereas they had occasionally been obscured in the thicker 5μ sections. In addition special stains could be used to demonstrate more clearly certain components in the renal biopsy.

Staining a 3μ section from a renal biopsy

Four staining techniques are commonly applied to renal biopsies: the haematoxylin and eosin stain, the periodic acid Schiff reaction, the Jones methenamine silver method and the Congo red stain for amyloid.

HAEMATOXYLIN AND EOSIN

This is a useful all-round stain but is less useful for detecting subtle abnormalities in the glomerulus than the PAS and methenamine silver stains. It is important, however, for the general assessment of tubules, hypercellularity, interstitium and blood vessels, and should never be neglected.

PERIODIC ACID SCHIFF REACTION

This stain is the best stain of glomerular capillary basement membranes that exists. In our opinion it remains so despite recent pressure from advocates of the Jones methenamine silver stain. Capillary basement membrane thickening of all degrees of severity can usually be detected with ease by this method (cf. Jones methenamine silver). Almost equally important is the fact that the mesangium of the glomerular tuft, in particular the acellular mesangial material, is well demonstrated by this stain (Fig. 10.1) and minor degrees of mesangial increase can easily be seen. The basement membranes

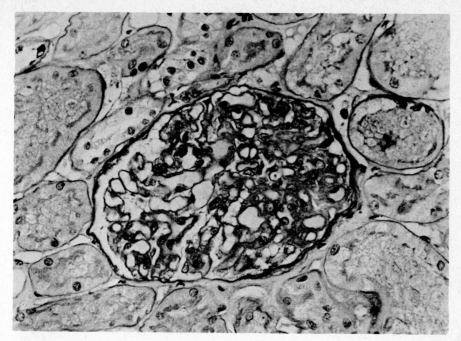

Figure 10.1 A 3μ paraffin section of a renal biopsy stained by the PAS reaction, showing segmental mesangial proliferation and basement membrane thickening. Magnification (× 392)

of the tubules are also well stained by the PAS method, but this is rarely of diagnostic importance.

JONES METHENAMINE SILVER STAIN

This attractive silver deposition method is a most useful stain in renal biopsies. It produces its best results when the tissue has been fixed in Bouin's fluid; fixation in formalin or paraformaldehyde may mean that the section will require a longer incubation in the methenamine silver than is given in the method below. Where fixation has only been for a short time the difference is hardly significant, but specimens which have been standing in formalin for a week or two may need a much longer staining time. Staining is preferably done under microscopic control, examining the section every 30 minutes or so, until the capillary basement membranes and glomerular mesangial material are stained brown. Note that the basement membranes of the tubules seem to stain earlier than those in glomerular tuft, so these are not a suitable 'end-point'.

The methenamine silver method nicely picks out the glomerular capillary basement membrane and the acellular mesangial material component of the mesangium, in a similar manner to the PAS reaction (Fig. 10.2). Our own feeling is that as a mesangial stain it is superior to the PAS, but as a basement membrane stain it is slightly inferior. The method gained its reputation as the best capillary basement membrane stain on its ability to demonstrate argyrophilic 'spikes' on the outer surface of the thickened basement membrane in membranous nephropathy. So popular did this concept become that for a time pathologists were almost afraid to diagnose membranous nephropathy

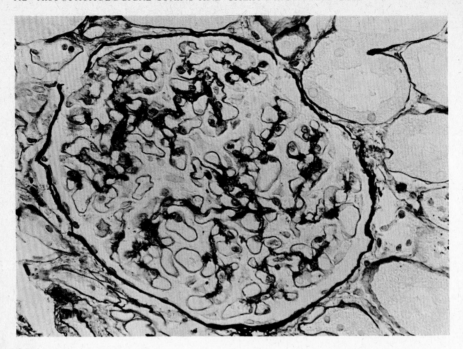

Figure 10.2 A 3μ paraffin section of a renal biopsy from a child with the nephrotic syndrome, stained by Jones methenamine silver method. The glomerular basement membranes and mesangial material stain black; in this glomerulus both are normal. The kidney was normal by light microscopy ('minimal change nephropathy'). (Magnification ($\times$ 252)

unless they were able to demonstrate spikes on the methenamine silver stained section. With the wider application of electron microscopical investigation of renal biopsies, however, it soon became apparent that 'spikes' were only present at certain stages in the gradual development of membranous nephropathy, and that not all the components of the steadily thickening basement membrane were argyrophilic. It is conceivable therefore that one may fail to detect a thickened basement membrane on the methenamine silver section, but pick it up with ease on the PAS section. For this reason the PAS reaction is the method of choice for glomerular basement membranes in 3μ sections. The most informative counterstain for use with the silver method is a light haematoxylin and eosin stain, rather than the light green counterstain recommended by most textbooks.

Congo Red Stain for Amyloid

The staining of amyloid is discussed in some detail in Chapter 5. In some instances amyloid can be detected easily on the H & E stained section, but occasionally minor degrees of amyloid involvement can only be detected by using a special amyloid stain. This occurs particularly in the odd case when the disease involves mainly the walls of vessels in the interstitium, whilst the pathologist's eyes seem magnetically attracted to the more glamorous glomeruli. There are two further advantages of routine Congo red staining of renal biopsies:

(i) the characteristic casts of Bence Jones light chain in the 'myeloma kidney' have the staining reactions of amyloid, and

(ii) the mere presence of a Congo red stained section on the slide tray is a constant reminder to the pathologist never to forget the possibility of amyloid.

These four stains are the basic tools of the renal pathologist's trade; other stains which are occasionally useful are:

ELASTIC VAN GIESON STAIN

This is useful in two main situations. First, in a hypertensive kidney, it emphasises the increase in number of the elastic lamellae in the internal elastic lamina; the van Gieson component of the stain also helps in assessing the muscular and intimal components of the vessel walls in hypertension. Secondly, this stain is useful in biopsies of renal transplants, where breaks in the internal elastic lamina in vessels usually imply a past episode of transplant rejection.

THE MSB STAIN

This trichrome method was developed by Lendrum et al (1962) to demonstrate fibrin, and as an attempt to differentiate between fibrin of differing ages. Its main application in renal biopsies is in the demonstration of 'fibrinoid' necrosis in arterioles or glomerular tufts (as in polyarteritis nodosa, scleroderma kidney, lupus nephritis and malignant hypertension), and in fibrin plugging of glomerular capillaries as in some cases of the haemolytic–uraemic syndrome. Fibrin can usually be easily distinguished on the H & E, but the MSB is useful in doubtful cases and, furthermore, is aesthetically pleasing and photographs superbly!

THE METHYL GREEN-PYRONIN (Unna–Pappenheim)

This stain demonstrates RNA in cell cytoplasm and is useful in biopsies of renal transplants. In transplants one of the changes seen in rejection is the aggregation around blood vessels of large lymphocyte-type cells, many of which have demonstrable RNA in their cytoplasm. The Unna–Pappenheim method stains the cytoplasm of these cells bright pink, as it does plasma cell cytoplasm.

Toluidine blue staining of 1μ sections

A recent advance in renal biopsy interpretation has followed the development of a method by which sections in the region of 1μ thick can be prepared. Paraffin wax offers inadequate support to the tissue block for this purpose, and the tissues are therefore embedded in a resin such as araldite or epon. The tissue is first fixed in glutaraldehyde, post-fixed in osmium tetroxide, dehydrated in ethanol, embedded in resin and the blocks are cut at 1μ on a pyramitome or ultramicrotome using glass knives. The sections are stained with toluidine blue. Much more information can be gleaned from renal biopsies in this way, in particular a far better assessment of basement membrane thickness, marginal mesangial increase and glomerular cellularity can be made. In addition, the various types of deposits in the basement membrane in such conditions as acute poststreptococcal glomerulonephritis, membranous nephropathy and lupus nephritis are easily seen by this technique (Fig. 10.3).

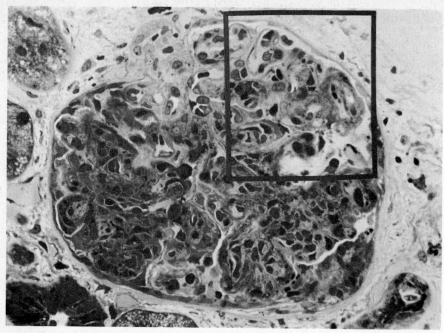

Figure 10.3 (a) A glomerulus in a toluidine blue-stained araldite-embedded 1 μ section of a renal biopsy from a man with lupus nephritis. The hypercellularity and dark-staining basement membrane deposits can be seen. Magnification (× 392)

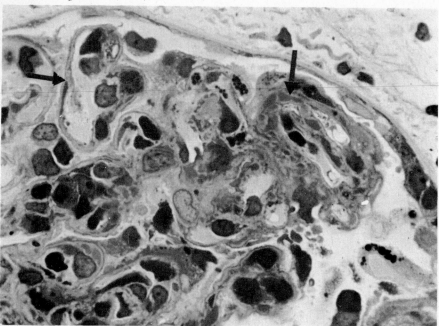

(b) A higher power view of the boxed area in (a) showing large intramembranous deposits (arrowed on the right). Compare with the more normal basement membrane on the left (arrowed) which contains an early subendothelial deposit only. Magnification (× 1008)

A useful ploy is to prepare high power, well-focused photomicrograph transparencies of the glomerulus under study and to project on to a screen. If there is no urgency to report the biopsy, this is the ideal way of getting the maximum information from a $1\,\mu$ section.

The great disadvantage of this method is that only a couple of glomeruli can be studied since the original block must be small, so there is a danger that a non-representative sample is examined. This is particularly important in focal renal lesions. However, progress is being made in preparing whole biopsy cores in araldite and cutting them at $1\,\mu$ using a broad glass knife. It is probable that eventually all renal biopsies will be treated in this way, and that paraffin-embedded $3\,\mu$ sections will become redundant. Another great advantage of this method is that relevant parts of the same araldite-embedded biopsy core can then be examined electron microscopically after trimming.

The toluidine blue method is the best staining technique to use in $1\,\mu$ araldite-embedded sections. Attempts to apply the stains used in $3\,\mu$ paraffin sections e.g. the Jones methenamine silver, are unsatisfactory and, even when successful, provide less information than the toluidine blue stain. A softer resin, 2-ethoxyethyl methacrylate, may be used. Specialised fixation is not necessary and sections can be cut at about $1\,\mu$ using a base sledge microtome and a well-sharpened knife. The PAS and Jones methenamine silver stains can be applied.

A summary of stains is given in Table 10.1.

Table 10.1. Renal biopsies—useful stains

Staining method	Abbreviation	Demonstrates	Page
Haematoxylin and eosin	H & E	General morphology	7
Martius-scarlet-blue	MSB	Fibrin, basement membranes, collagen	45
Weigert's elastic	LEHVG	Elastic fibres	43
Verhoeff's elastic	VE	Elastic fibres	46
Periodic acid Schiff	PAS	Basement membranes, mesangium	19
Methenamine silver	(PA)MS	Basement membranes, mesangium	118
Congo red	CR	Amyloid, myeloma casts	56
Toluidine blue	TB	Detailed morphology, basement membrane deposits	118
Methyl green pyronin	UP	Plasma cells, 'immunoblasts'	119

Fixation

Bouin's fluid is the fixative of choice for paraffin-embedded $3\,\mu$ sections, although formol saline may be used. Glutaraldehyde is the fixative of choice for toluidine blue-stained $1\,\mu$ araldite-embedded sections. A useful compromise is paraformaldehyde, which can be used as a fixative for both paraffin and resin embedding; it gives less perfect preservation for electron microscopy than glutaraldehyde, and the Jones methenamine silver $3\,\mu$ paraffin section may need longer in the silver stain than the recommended time, but it is a most useful all-round fixative where the ultimate fate of the biopsy material is not known.

Urgent biopsies

In some cases the result of a renal biopsy will be required within 24 hours, e.g. in acute renal failure of unknown aetiology. In this instance the needle biopsy is treated differently and processed as below.

1. Upon receipt in the laboratory, place biopsy in fresh, warm Carnoy's fixative at 56°C for 45 minutes to 1 hour.
2. Transfer to absolute alcohol and chloroform 1:1 at 56°C for 1 hour.
3. Transfer to chloroform at 56°C for 15 minutes.
4. Transfer to fresh chloroform at 56°C for 30 minutes.
5. Transfer to paraffin wax for 15 minutes.
6. Transfer to fresh wax for 30 minutes.
7. Transfer to fresh wax for 45 minutes.
8. Embed in fresh wax.

PREPARATION OF RENAL BIOPSIES FOR THIN SECTIONING

The technique given here allows thin 1μ sections to be cut, suitable for toluidine blue staining. It also allows the same material to be used for electron microscopy if facilities are available.

The biopsy specimen should be treated with great care. It is usually advisable for a member of the technical staff to collect the specimen immediately after removal from the patient. The specimen is placed into saline and examined under a dissecting microscope. A piece approximately 3 mm long, containing glomeruli, is cut from the specimen and placed in glutaraldehyde fixative. The remainder of the biopsy is processed for conventional histology.

SOLUTIONS

1. *Primary fixative: glutaraldehyde*

2.26 per cent sodium dihydrogen orthophosphate ($NaH_2PO_4.2H_2O$)	83 ml
2.52 per cent sodium hydroxide	17 ml
0.1M calcium chloride	0.5 ml
Sucrose	3 g
25 per cent glutaraldehyde	3 ml

To the sodium dihydrogen orthophosphate add the sodium hydroxide, check pH and adjust to 7.3–7.4 if necessary. Add the calcium chloride solution drop by drop and agitate solution. Add sufficient of this solution to the sucrose to make the total 100 ml. To 22 ml of this solution add the glutaraldehyde to make the working fixative (which should be prepared fresh daily).

2. *Buffer wash*

2.26 per cent sodium dihydrogen orthophosphate ($NaH_2PO_4.2H_2O$)	83 ml
2.52 per cent sodium hydroxide	17 ml
0.1M calcium chloride	0.5 ml
Sucrose	5 g

To the sodium dihydrogen orthophosphate add the sodium hydroxide, check pH and adjust to 7.3–7.4 if necessary. Add the calcium chloride drop by drop and agitate, then add sufficient of this solution to the sucrose to make the total 100 ml.

3. *Post-fixative*

4.52 per cent sodium dihydrogen orthophosphate ($NaH_2PO_4.2H_2O$)	20.75 ml
5.04 per cent sodium hydroxide	4.25 ml
0.2M calcium chloride	1 drop
Sucrose	250 mg
2 per cent aqueous osmium tetroxide	5 ml

To the sodium dihydrogen orthophosphate add the sodium hydroxide and 1 drop of calcium chloride. Shake, check pH is 7.2, if not adjust. Add sufficient of this solution to the sucrose to make the volume 12.5 ml. For the working solution add aqueous osmium tetroxide to 5 ml of the solution.

4. *Epoxypropane–resin solution*

Araldite CY212	25 ml
HY964 hardener	25 ml
DY064 accelerator	0.75 ml
1:2 epoxypropane	50 ml

5. *Pure resin solution*

Araldite CY212	25 ml
HY964 hardener	25 ml
DY064 accelerator	0.75 ml

6. *Toluidine blue staining solution*

Sodium tetraborate (borax)	1 g
Distilled water	120 ml
Pyronin Y	0.2 g
Toluidine blue	1.0 g

Dissolve the sodium tetraborate in the distilled water, before adding the two dyes. Filter before use.

FIXATION METHOD
1. Place the tissue in a bijou bottle containing 3 per cent glutaraldehyde (solution 1) for 2 hours at 4°C.
2. Wash in buffer solution (solution 2), three changes of 30 minutes each at 4°C (the tissue may also be left in this solution overnight).
3. Post-fix in 1 per cent osmium tetroxide (solution 3) for 1 hour at 4°C followed by 30 minutes at room temperature.
4. Rinse in distilled water.

DEHYDRATION METHOD (performed at room temperature)
1. Following the rinse in distilled water, place in 50 per cent alcohol for 15 minutes.
2. 70 per cent alcohol for 15 minutes.
3. 95 per cent alcohol for 15 minutes.
4. Absolute alcohol, previously filtered through anhydrous sodium sulphate, for 30 minutes.
5. Fresh change of absolute alcohol, filtered as above, for 30 minutes.

EMBEDDING METHOD
1. Following treatment with absolute alcohol place the tissue in 1:2 epoxy-propane for 20 minutes.
2. A further change of 1:2 epoxypropane for 20 minutes.
3. Place in epoxypropane–resin mixture (solution 4) for 1 hour.
4. Leave in pure resin overnight (solution 5) in uncapped vials at room temperature.
5. Infiltrate with fresh resin at 60°C, two changes of 30 minutes each. After each change rotate the vials to ensure contact of the tissue with fresh resin.
6. Embed the tissue in warm resin at 60°C in Taab capsules (Taab Laboratories Ltd, Reading) and polymerise for 48 hours at 60°C.

CUTTING AND STAINING
   One micron sections can be cut on an ultramicrotome, an LKB pyramitome or on a modified base sledge. These sections are picked up on glass slides and dried at a high temperature (70°C) on a hot plate. Staining is carried out using toluidine blue at 70°C (solution 6) for 30 seconds to 1 minute, followed by a rinse in hot tap water, blot and then dried at room temperature before mounting in DPX. For other tissues it may be necessary to increase the staining time.

STAINING METHODS

Methenamine Silver (Jones, 1957)
   This silver solution is used to demonstrate many substances, i.e. urates, fungi, mucin and basement membranes. The method depends upon the oxidation of 1:2 glycol groups to produce free aldehydes; these in turn reduce the silver solution to produce the silver precipitate on the glomerular capillary and tubular basement membranes.

SOLUTIONS

Stock silver solution

3 per cent aqueous hexamine	100 ml
5 per cent silver nitrate in distilled water	5 ml

To the 3 per cent hexamine add the 5 per cent silver nitrate (in distilled water). A precipitate will form. Continue to shake until this precipitate clears. Store at 4°C.

Working solution (prepare freshly)

Silver solution	25 ml
Distilled water	20 ml
Boric acid	160 mg
Sodium tetraborate	130 mg

METHOD
1. Place sections in xylol, then down to water.
2. Place in 0.5 per cent periodic acid for 15 minutes.
3. Wash in tap water.
4. Wash well in distilled water.
5. Place in hexamine silver solution for 2–3 hours at 50°C.
6. Wash in distilled water.
7. Tone in 0.2 per cent gold chloride for 1 minute (until brown staining turns black).
8. Fix in 3 per cent sodium thiosulphate for 2 minutes.
9. Wash in running tap water for 5 minutes.
10. Counterstain in 1 per cent light green or counterstain with a very light haematoxylin and eosin.
11. Wash in tap water.
12. Dehydrate, clear and mount.

RESULTS
Basement membranes and mesangial material: *black.*

NOTES
1. Thin sections of 1–3 μ to be used.
2. The time required in the silver solution varies according to fixative used. Formaldehyde and paraformaldehyde fixed tissues will need longer than Bouin-fixed material. Tissues that have been in fixative for more than a few days may need longer in the silver solution, and staining will probably be less precise.
3. Tubular basement membranes stain earlier than glomerular capillary basement membranes. Ensure when checking microscopically after stage 5 that silver precipitation has occurred on glomerular capillary basement membranes.

Methyl green pyronin method (Unna–Pappenheim)
   This technique is capable of demonstrating both RNA and DNA. The technique was first used by Pappenheim in 1899. It was improved in 1902 by Unna who added phenol, and it is therefore commonly known as the Unna–Pappenheim method; because of the two dyes used it is also known as the methyl green pyronin method. The method uses two basic dyes, methyl green and pyronin, both of which are impure stains; methyl green always contains methyl violet which must be removed by washing in chloroform. Methyl green is not specific for DNA but it is highly selective if washed and used at a slightly acid pH. Pyronin is not specific for RNA except when used with suitable extraction methods. As can be seen, pH is very important; at very acid pH levels methyl green will not stain, whereas at alkaline pH

pyronin works poorly. To obtain good RNA and DNA staining the two dyes should be used in a solution with a pH of 4.8. The method tends to be capricious and three factors seem important: (a) fixation, neutral formalin or alcohol giving the best results, (b) some batches of pyronin Y fail to give satisfactory results, (c) correct pH.

SOLUTIONS

Methyl green

Methyl green	2 g
Distilled water	100 ml

When dissolved the methyl green is washed with equal quantities of chloroform until no violet colour is seen in the chloroform; this will take five or six washes. Store over fresh chloroform.

Pyronin Y

Pyronin Y	2 g
Distilled water	100 ml

This solution is washed five or six times with chloroform as described above and stored over fresh chloroform.

Buffer solution

Sodium acetate	41 mg
Glacial acetic acid (concentrated)	0.3 ml
Distilled water	50.0 ml

Staining solution: methyl green pyronin

Methyl green	7.5 ml
Pyronin Y	12.5 ml
Buffer	30.0 ml

METHOD
1. Place sections in xylol, then down to water.
2. Rinse in distilled water, blot dry.
3. Stain in methyl green pyronin solution for 20 minutes.
4. Rinse rapidly in tap water, then blot.
5. Rinse in acetone for 30–45 seconds.
6. Rinse in acetone–xylol 1 : 1 for 30 seconds.
7. Clear in xylol and mount.

RESULTS
DNA, e.g. nuclei: *green* or *blue-green*.
RNA, plasma cell cytoplasm: *red, pink*.

NOTES
1. For precise results extraction techniques for RNA and DNA must be used (see p. 17).
2. Acid fixatives should be avoided.

REFERENCES

JONES, D. B. (1957). Nephrotic glomerulonephritis. *Amer. J. Path.,* **33,** 313.

LENDRUM, A. C., FRASER, D. S., SLIDDERS, W. & HENDERSON, R. (1962). Studies on the character and staining of fibrin. *J. clin. Path.,* **15,** 401.

PAPPENHEIM, A. (1899). Vergleischende untersuchungen uber die elementare Zusammensetzung des rothen knockenmarkes einiger Saugethiere. *Virchows Arch. path. Anat.,* **157,** 19.

UNNA, P. G. (1902). Eine modifikation der Pappenheimschen Farbung auf granoplasma. *Mh. prakt. Derm.,* **35,** 76.

FURTHER READING

CLAYDEN, E. C. (1971). *Practical Section Cutting and Staining,* 5th edition. Edinburgh & London: Churchill Livingstone.

HEPTINSTALL, R. N. (1966). *Pathology of the Kidney.* London: Churchill.

MEADOWS, R. (1973). *Renal Histopathology—A Light Microscopic Study of Renal Disease.* Oxford University Press.

CHAPTER 11

Other Specialised Biopsies

LIVER BIOPSIES

Liver biopsies are received in one of two forms, either as a narrow, fragile core of tissue 2 mm across and 10 mm long, removed by closed needle biopsy, or as a more substantial wedge of tissue removed at laparotomy. The needle biopsy core requires delicate handling, and particular care must be taken during wax embedding to ensure that the core is embedded absolutely flat so that full longitudinal sections can be cut. If the embedding or orientation are slightly awry, potentially valuable pieces of an already small specimen may be lost in the preliminary trimming of the block. Despite its small size a needle biopsy core usually gives a reasonable picture of what is going on in the liver, but of course isolated tumours such as a liver cell carcinoma may be missed. Another sampling problem arises when the liver shows severe cirrhosis with thick fibrous bands; here the needle tends to ricochet off the hard fibrous tissue and to bore only through the softer parenchymal tissue, producing a non-representative specimen which understates the severity of the fibrosis. A similar situation arises in occasional cases where the liver is packed with metastatic tumour, particularly where the tumour nodules have a strong fibrous stroma (as in some cases of carcinoma of the breast); again the needle has a tendency to slide in the soft liver parenchyma between tumour nodules.

In many respects the wedge biopsy is better than a needle biopsy, since a larger specimen is obtained and the surgeon can select the most abnormal area, so solitary tumours are less likely to be missed. However, for reasons of convenience and haemostasis the surgeon usually removes the wedge from the lower margin of the anterior part of the liver, and this produces an important pitfall for the unwary pathologist. At the anterior inferior border of the liver the architecture of the liver's lobular pattern is distorted: the fibrous septa running from the liver capsule to the subcapsular portal triads are thick, split liver lobules, and often run to the central veins. The portal triads themselves may show increased fibrous tissue and bile duct reduplication. All these features may suggest cirrhosis to the inexperienced eye. Furthermore, there may be clumps of neutrophils underneath the liver capsule and within the liver parenchyma; in these circumstances this finding is of no significance and is usually seen when the wedge biopsy is performed towards the end of a laparotomy, particularly when there has been much handling of the viscera.

Processing

The small needle biopsy may be processed manually during a working day with a four to six-hour schedule. The wedge biopsy should be processed on the tissue processor in the normal way.

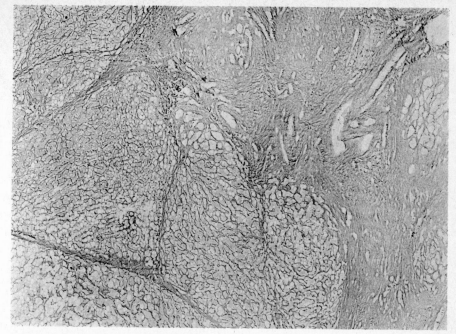

Figure 11.1 Liver biopsy from a patient with cirrhosis. The reticulin stain (Gordon and Sweet) emphasises the fibrosis and disruption of the liver's lobular architecture. Magnification (× 40)

Sectioning

The sectioning of a needle biopsy must be done with great care. As the biopsy is so thin it is advisable to cut serial sections to cover all possible needs, usually about 12 sections. For a laboratory doing liver needle biopsies as a routine, the following procedures may be found helpful:

Section 1. H & E
2. Reticulin stain
3. Perls' stain for iron
4. PAS (or Best's carmine)
5. Van Gieson
6. Long ZN, Schmorl, or Sudan black for lipofuscin.

This leaves six sections for other stains (e.g. Congo red, elastic van Gieson, MSB) should the need arise.

Staining methods

Haematoxylin and eosin for general morphology.

Reticulin stain (Gordon and Sweet, 1936) to demonstrate the reticulin network and to emphasise any abnormality of the hepatic architecture (Fig. 11.1). This stain is particularly useful to detect minor degrees of cirrhotic change and to pinpoint foci of liver cell necrosis or atrophy, as in infective hepatitis.

Iron stain (Perls, 1967) to detect excessive amounts of iron and its distribution, as in haemochromatosis or transfusional siderosis.

In addition the following stains may be useful:

PAS reaction and *Best's carmine* for detection of glycogen.

Van Gieson stain, a fine stain for collagen, useful in cirrhosis or scarring of all degrees of severity. An added bonus is that van Gieson's stain is a useful and convenient way of demonstrating bile, which it stains green.

Long Ziehl–Neelsen, a good stain for the positive identification of lipofuscin and its differentiation from haemosiderin and other pigments.

Electron microscopy and thin sections

It is inevitable that within the next few years electron microscopy will become increasingly used in the diagnosis of some liver diseases, and will eventually play as big a role as it does today in renal biopsy interpretation. A small piece of the fresh needle biopsy core is removed with a sharp scalpel blade and fixed in buffered glutaraldehyde for subsequent araldite embedding (see p. 116).

For those laboratories without facilities for electron microscopy much information can be obtained from some liver biopsies by the preparation of $1\,\mu$ sections of glutaraldehyde-fixed araldite-embedded tissues stained by the toluidine blue method. The techniques are identical to those described in Chapter 10. The special equipment needed is an ultratome, pyramitome or a modified base-sledge microtome to cut the $1\,\mu$ sections. Ultra-thin sections can subsequently be prepared from the araldite block using an ultratome, and more detailed ultrastructural changes noted with the electron microscope.

Paraformaldehyde is a suitable compromise as a first fixative for the whole biopsy specimen since it is suitable for either subsequent paraffin or araldite embedding and gives sufficiently good tissue preservation to make electron microscopy worthwhile.

Frozen sections

Frozen sections for rapid diagnosis of liver disease are rarely indicated, particularly since a needle biopsy specimen can be rapidly processed and a paraffin section obtained within 6 hours. The only absolute indication for frozen section is in the diagnosis of lipid and glycogen storage diseases; an open wedge biopsy is preferable since, from a practical point of view, the preparation of good cryostat sections from a needle biopsy specimen may be difficult because of problems with orientation.

A summary of staining methods is given in Table 11.1.

Table 11.1. Staining methods for liver biopsies

Staining method	Application	See page
Periodic acid Schiff	Glycogen and other PAS-positive material	19
Best's carmine	Glycogen	128
Bauer–Feulgen	Glycogen in frozen sections	130
Perls'	Ferric iron	87
Weigert's elastic	Elastic tissue	43
Schmorl	Lipofuscin, melanin	88
Long ZN	Lipofuscin	92
Sudan black	Lipofuscin	32
Reticulin stain	Reticulin network	41
MSB	Fibrin, collagen	45
Congo red	Amyloid	56

TESTICULAR BIOPSIES

Testicular biopsy is performed mainly in the investigation of male infertility. The many possible testicular causes for aspermia and oligospermia can be differentiated histologically, so that the potentially treatable testicular abnormalities (e.g. tubular blockage associated with varicocoele) can be treated. Testicular biopsy is ill-advised where a testicular tumour is suspected clinically because of the dangers of tumour dissemination. The biopsy specimen is obtained by making a small nick in the scrotum and a similar nick through the tunica until light brown testicular tissue bulges out; a small piece is gently snipped off and placed in fixative. Formol saline, formol sublimate or Bouin's fluid are all suitable fixatives, and a haematoxylin and eosin stain is usually all that is required, although a van Gieson stain gives a more accurate demonstration of any interstitial fibrosis. The nuclear changes in disordered spermatogenesis are elegantly demonstrated by a properly performed Heidenhain's iron haematoxylin stain, although this is a tedious chore for the technologist and an unnecessary self-indulgence for the pathologist.

The biopsy should be processed in such a manner as to produce as little shrinkage as possible. Artefacts may be produced if the floating-out bath for the sections is too warm, as the section will lose its normal pattern.

JEJUNAL BIOPSIES

Jejunal biopsy is performed where there is suspicion of disease in the small intestine, particularly where there is evidence of malabsorption of food, as in 'coeliac' disease (gluten enteropathy). The biopsy specimen is obtained by a Crosby capsule, a device which is swallowed by the patient and which snips off a piece of jejunal mucosa and submucosa; the capsule is then withdrawn and the biopsy specimen removed.

Laboratory handling

Jejunal biopsy specimens must be handled with the utmost care. In laboratories where this biopsy is reasonably common a standard procedure is followed. On removal, the biopsy specimen is placed in cold (4°C) formol calcium and viewed under the dissecting microscope, mucosa upwards; the number, height and shape of the villi are noted and the specimen is photographed if possible. The specimen is then treated in one of two ways:

FOR ROUTINE HISTOLOGY

The specimen is arranged flat on a piece of card with the mucosa straightened and the villi vertical, and allowed to fix in formol calcium or formol saline at room temperature. Processing of the biopsy is by a short daytime schedule, to minimise shrinkage. Great care must be taken with the orientation of the specimen at the embedding stage, for the wrong positioning of the specimen can nullify the whole procedure. Few special staining methods are required for these biopsies, an H & E and an acid mucosubstance method usually being sufficient.

FOR ENZYME AND OTHER HISTOCHEMISTRY

The demonstration of hydrolytic enzymes may be informative and, to this end, fixation of the specimen is continued overnight in formol calcium at 4°C, followed by treatment in gum sucrose and subsequent sectioning in a cryostat. Again correct orientation of the specimen is vital. Demonstration of oxidative enzymes is not usually possible in fixed material.

RECTAL BIOPSIES

Rectal biopsy may be performed for a number of reasons: for the diagnosis of rectal tumours, inflammatory diseases of the rectum and for the diagnosis of systematised amyloidosis. Accurate orientation of the specimen is again vital; it should be placed on to a piece of card before fixation in formol saline. At the embedding stage care must be taken that the orientation is correct so that a section will include mucosa, submucosa, and any muscle without obliquity.

For the diagnosis of neoplastic and inflammatory conditions an H & E is usually all that is necessary, although a mucin stain such as alcian blue may be helpful in such conditions as ulcerative colitis and adenocarcinoma.

For the diagnosis of amyloid the stains and techniques described in Chapter 5 are applied. Although the detection of small amounts of amyloid is facilitated by applying the Congo red technique to frozen sections, it is rarely worth risking possible loss of a small and valuable biopsy specimen for a marginal increase in detection rate.

Rectal or colonic biopsy is occasionally performed in suspected Hirschsprung's disease, the diagnosis being based on the absence of ganglion cells from the plexus between the layers of the muscularis and in the sub-mucosa. Occasionally biopsies are performed during an operation for resection of the affected aganglionic segment so that it can be completely excised. Cryostat sections are prepared and stained, usually with H & E or methylene blue, to demonstrate the presence or absence of ganglion cells. Numerous enzyme histochemical methods (e.g. non-specific esterase) have been advocated to facilitate the rapid detection of ganglion cells, but the adequacy of the specimen and its correct orientation are as important as the staining method used.

MUSCLE BIOPSIES

Biopsy of striated muscle is performed in patients with muscle weakness, tenderness or atrophy in an attempt to determine the underlying pathology. The histological appearances enable the pathologist to distinguish between myopathy, myositis, denervation, etc. A fruitful muscle biopsy depends on collaboration between the physician, who will indicate which accessible muscle is most likely to show pathological changes, the surgeon, who will excise an adequate specimen from the chosen muscle with care and gentleness, and the pathologist who will prepare and examine the specimen using all the means at his disposal. It is advisable to maintain the muscle at stretch from the outset, so it is helpful if the surgeon ties each end of the biopsy specimen before excision and maintains tension on the silks throughout. A useful manoeuvre is for the surgeon to tie the piece of muscle to be removed to either end of a piece of orange stick before excision; this maintains the muscle biopsy at the correct tension and allows neither shrinkage nor over-stretching.

Fixation

A small piece of muscle is fixed in glutaraldehyde for possible electron miscroscopy or 1μ sections, and a larger unfixed piece (up to $4 \times 4 \times 3$ mm) is frozen in liquid nitrogen after being allowed to stand in a moist atmosphere (i.e. on moist filter paper in a closed petri dish). This last manoeuvre prevents sudden contraction of the muscle on freezing. Isopentane or arcton can be used with the liquid nitrogen, as these gases produce a higher rate of thermal conductivity and consequently a faster rate of freezing. This frozen specimen is for histochemistry; sectioning of muscle biopsies in the cryostat presents no problem providing the temperature is maintained below $-18°C$. It is essential that the frozen specimen is orientated in such a way that the sections show the muscle fibres cut transversely.

As soon as the main muscle biopsy specimen has been removed it is pinned on a flat piece of card or cork at its original tension, and is left in a moist atmosphere for 30 minutes or so before fixation. Fixation is by 10 per cent neutral formol saline, formol calcium or formol sublimate for 24 hours, still pinned out on the card. After fixation the biopsy specimen is cut into two pieces with a sharp scalpel blade to produce two blocks, one which can be cut to provide transverse sections of muscle fibres and the other to be cut to show the fibres in longitudinal section. Muscle biopsies should always receive adequate fixation and slow careful processing for the most successful results; large pieces of muscle should be double embedded.

Staining methods

The following methods are commonly used in muscle biopsies:

Haematoxylin and eosin for general morphology. In a well-performed H & E, regenerating muscle fibres can be detected because they are slightly more basophilic than normal fibres. The H & E also demonstrates the nature of any cellular infiltrate or vascular abnormalities.

Elastic van Gieson demonstrates collagen, and also picks up any abnormality of arterial elastica, e.g. in old arteritis, and stains the myelin of peripheral nerve endings. Some pathologists prefer a trichrome stain for these purposes. One advantage of the trichrome method is that it demonstrates the rods in nemaline myopathy.

Unna–Pappenheim (Unna, 1902; Pappenheim, 1899) emphasises any regenerating muscle fibres. These have a high RNA content and are more pyroninophilic than normal fibres. Nemaline rods stain deeply red by this method.

PAS reaction demonstrates any glycogen in muscle fibres; positive identification of glycogen depends upon the disappearance of PAS positivity after pretreatment with diastase.

Enzyme histochemical methods

Many enzyme histochemical methods have been applied to cryostat sections of muscle biopsies. The three given below are probably the most widely used and generally informative.

Succinate dehydrogenase (SDH) enables Type 1 and Type 2 fibres to be distinguished: Type 1 fibres stain darkly and Type 2 stain lightly by this method. Other enzymes of the oxidative cycle have similar reactions.

Muscle adenosine triphosphatase (ATPase) also enables Type 1 and Type 2 fibres to be distinguished, although this time Type 1 fibres stain weakly and Type 2 fibres strongly. The enzyme method is usually performed at a pH of 9.4; if the tissue is preincubated at pH 4.6 some of the fibres subsequently stain differently. On the basis of this, and certain other enzyme reactions, the Type 2 fibres have been subdivided into Types 2A, 2B and 2C.

Phosphorylase also enables the two different fibre types to be distinguished, but less clearly than the two methods mentioned above, since some fibres stain with intermediate intensity. Its value lies in its application to the phosphorylase deficiency myopathy, McArdle's disease.

The value of the enzyme methods is in their ability to distinguish between the two basic types of muscle fibres; the variations in size, number and distribution of the two fibre types may have considerable diagnostic importance.

Electron microscopy

Electron microscopy may be of vital importance in the diagnosis of certain rare myopathies, and is of confirmatory value in other muscle diseases, although very many of the ultrastructural abnormalities are completely non-specific and the same changes can be seen in a wide variety of different muscle diseases.

STAINING METHODS

Best's carmine method for glycogen (Best, 1906)

This technique, when used alongside diastase digestion, appears to be specific for glycogen although the staining mechanism is not known.

SOLUTIONS

Best's carmine stock solution

Carmine (Best)	2 g
Potassium carbonate	1 g
Potassium chloride	5 g
Distilled water	60 ml
Ammonia (.880)	20 ml

Boil first four ingredients gently for 5 minutes, cool and filter. Add the ammonia and store at 4°C.

Working solution

Stock solution	10 ml
Ammonia (.880)	15 ml
Methyl alcohol	15 ml

Best's differentiator

Absolute alcohol	40 ml
Methyl alcohol	20 ml
Distilled water	50 ml

METHOD
1. Place sections in xylol, then down to water.
2. Stain sections in celestin blue for 5 minutes.
3. Wash in water.
4. Stain in haematoxylin for 5 minutes.
5. Wash in tap water for 5 minutes.
6. Stain in Best's carmine working solution for 15 minutes.
7. Differentiate in Best's differentiator for 1–3 minutes.
8. Transfer to absolute alcohol.
9. Place in xylol and mount in DPX.

RESULTS
Glycogen: *bright red.*
Nuclei: *blue.*

NOTES
1. The original method advises that celloidin sections be used to avoid the diffusion of glycogen; later, celloidin-coated paraffin sections were used for the same reason. There is no need to celloidinise the sections unless there is a danger of them lifting off in the alkaline staining solution.
2. The glycogen-staining solution will remove the haematoxylin from the section if left on for too long.
3. The staining solution deteriorates after two months at 4°C.
4. Not all batches of stain work satisfactorily.

Diastase method (for removal of glycogen in sections)
The method given below can be applied to any of the glycogen-demonstration methods. It will remove only glycogen of the relevant mucosubstances.

METHOD
1. Place sections in xylol, then down to water.
2. Treat with 0.1 per cent malt diastase in distilled water for 30 minutes.
3. Wash well in running tap water.
4. Stain alongside an untreated section with the glycogen method to be used.

RESULT
Any material positive in the untreated section and negative in the treated section can be assumed to be glycogen.

NOTES
Saliva may be used in place of the commercial malt diastase and is probably more convenient for the occasional slide.

Bauer–Feulgen method for glycogen (Bauer, 1933)

This method satisfactorily demonstrates glycogen in frozen sections.

SOLUTIONS

Schiff's reagent
See page 19.

METHOD

1. Place fixed frozen sections in tap water.
2. Oxidase in 4 per cent chromic acid for 10 minutes.
3. Wash well in tap water.
4. Place in Schiff's reagent (see p. 19) for 15 minutes.
5. Wash in tap water.
6. Counterstain in Mayer's haemalum for 2–4 minutes.
7. Wash well in tap water.
8. Dehydrate, clear and mount in DPX.

RESULTS

Glycogen: *red.*
Nuclei: *blue.*

NOTES

1. Mucosubstances other than glycogen are over-oxidised by the chromic acid and will not stain.
2. A sulphurous acid rinse may be used after stage 4; this is optional.

Incubating method for phosphorylase (Lake, 1970)

Fresh unfixed cryostat sections must be used for the technique.

SOLUTIONS

Incubating solution (add in order given)

0.1M acetate buffer pH 5.0	10 ml
0.1M magnesium chloride	1 ml
Glucose-1-phosphate (dipotassium salt)	100 mg
Glycogen (rabbit liver)	2 mg
Adenosine-5-monophosphate	5 mg
Adenosine-5-triphosphate	5 mg
Sodium fluoride	180 mg
Ethyl alcohol	2 ml
PVP	900 mg

Use solution unfiltered. This solution may be prepared in advance and stored frozen at −20°C.

Dilute Lugol's iodine

Lugol's iodine	1 part
Distilled water	30 parts

METHOD
1. Cut cryostat sections 7μ thick.
2. Place in incubating solution for 1 hour at 37°C.
3. Wash sections in 40 per cent alcohol.
4. Air dry.
5. Fix in absolute alcohol for 3 minutes.
6. Air dry.
7. Place in dilute Lugol's iodine solution for 5 minutes.
8. Mount in glycerol 9 parts to 1 part Lugol's iodine.

RESULTS
Phosphorylase activity: *black*.

NOTES
   Fading takes place rapidly, sections must be looked at immediately. Reaction may be renewed by repeating steps 7 and 8.

Adenosine triphosphatase (ATPase)
   This histochemical method is normally carried out at the alkaline pH of 9.4. By changing the pH, different types of muscle fibres may be shown (Dubowitz and Brooke, 1973); this alteration of pH can be brought about by preincubation in acetate buffer. The method given below is the calcium method of Padykula and Herman (1955) as modified by Dubowitz and Brooke (1973).

SOLUTIONS
Buffer solution

0.1M sodium barbitone	2 ml
0.18M calcium chloride	2 ml
Distilled water	6 ml

Adjust pH to 9.4.

Incubating solution

0.1M sodium barbitone	2 ml
0.18M calcium chloride	1 ml
Distilled water	7 ml
ATP (disodium salt)	25 mg

Adjust to pH 9.4.

METHOD
1. Rinse sections in buffer solution for 15 minutes.
2. Place sections in incubating solution for 45 minutes at 37°C.
3. Wash in three changes of 1 per cent aqueous calcium chloride.
4. Transfer sections to 2 per cent aqueous cobalt chloride for 3 minutes.
5. Rinse in four changes of 0.01M sodium barbitone.
6. Rinse in tap water.
7. Transfer to 1 per cent ammonium sulphide for 20–30 seconds.
8. Rinse in tap water.
9. Dehydrate, clear and mount in DPX.

RESULTS
ATPase activity: *black*.

Succinate dehydrogenase (Pearse, 1960)
   Unfixed cryostat sections must be employed for this method.

SOLUTIONS

Sodium succinate solution

Sodium succinate	1.62 g
Distilled water	8.00 ml
N hydrochloric acid	0.05 ml

Dissolve the succinate in the distilled water and add to the HCl. Check the pH of the solution and adjust to pH 7.1 if necessary, then make volume up to 10 ml with distilled water. Keeps well if frozen.

Dehydrogenase stock solution

MTT* (1 mg/ml)	2.5 ml
Tris buffer (pH 7.4)	2.5 ml
0.5M cobalt chloride	0.5 ml
Distilled water	3.5 ml

Check pH and adjust to 7.0 if necessary using stock tris buffer or N–hydrochloric acid. Keeps well if frozen.

Final incubating solution

Succinate solution	0.1 ml
Dehydrogenase stock solution	0.9 ml

METHOD
1. Cut cryostat sections 7 μ thick.
2. Place in incubating solution for 45 minutes at 37°C.
3. Transfer sections to 10 per cent formol saline for 15 minutes.
4. Rinse in distilled water.
5. Counterstain in 2 per cent methyl green (chloroform washed) for 5 minutes.
6. Rinse in tap water.
7. Mount in glycerin jelly.

RESULTS
Succinate dehydrogenase: *black* formazan deposit.
Nuclei: *green*.

NOTES
   Stock dehydrogenase solution may be used for any of the dehydrogenase enzymes.

* 3(4,5-dimethyl thiazolyl-2)5-diphenyl tetrazolium bromide.

Table 11.2. Useful histological and histochemical methods for muscle biopsies

Method	Demonstrates	Page
Haematoxylin and eosin	General morphology	7
Elastic van Gieson	Elastic fibres	43
Masson's trichrome	Collagen, muscle	42
MSB	Collagen	45
Congo red	Amyloid	56
Succinate dehydrogenase	Types 1 and 2 fibres	132
Phosphorylase	McArdle's disease	130
PAS with diastase control	Glycogen	19
Methyl green pyronin	Regenerating muscle	119
ATPase	Types 1 and 2 fibres	131

REFERENCES

BAUER, H. (1933). Mikroskopisch-chemischer Nachweis von Glykagen und einigen andersen Polysacchariden. *Z. mikr.-anat. Forsch.*, **33**, 143.

BEST, F. (1906). Ueber Karminfarbung des Glykogens und der Kerne. *Z. wiss. Mikr.*, **23**, 319.

DUBOWITZ, V. & BROOKE, M. (1973). *Muscle Biopsy, A Modern Approach.* London: Saunders.

GORDON, H. & SWEET, H. H. (1936). A simple method for the silver impregnation of reticulin. *Amer. J. Path.*, **12**, 545.

LAKE, B. (1970). The histochemical evaluation of the storage diseases. A review of techniques and their limitations. *J. Histochem.*, **2**, 441.

PADYKULA, H. A. & HERMAN, E. (1955). The specificity of the histochemical method for adenosine triphosphatase. *J. Histochem. Cytochem.*, **3**, 170.

PAPPENHEIM, A. (1899). Vergleichende untersuchungen urber die elementare Zuzammensetzung des rothen knochen markes einger Saugethiere. *Virchows Arch. path. Anat.*, **157**, 19.

PEARSE, A. G. E. (1970). *Histochemistry, Theoretical and Applied*, Vol. 2. Edinburgh & London: Churchill Livingstone.

PERLS, M. (1867). Nachweis Von Eisenoxyd in gewissen pigmenten. *Virchows Arch. path. Anat.*, **39**, 42.

VAN GIESON, I. (1889). Laboratory notes of technical methods for the nervous system. *N.Y. med. J.*, **50**, 57.

UNNA, P. G. (1902). Eine Modifikation der pappenheimschen Färbung Auf Granoplasma. *Mh. prakt. Derm.*, **35**, 76.

FURTHER READING

BANCROFT, J. D. (1975). *An Introduction to Histochemical Technique*, 2nd edition. London: Butterworths (in Press).

CLAYDEN, E. C. (1971). *Practical Section Cutting and Staining.* Edinburgh & London: Churchill Livingstone.

DICK, A. P., LENNARD-JONES, J. E., HYWELL-JONES, J. & MORSON, B. C. (1970). Technique for suction biopsy of the rectal mucosa. *Gut*, **11**, 182–184.

GEAR, E. V. & DOBBINS, W. O. (1968). Rectal biopsy: A review of its diagnostic usefulness. *Gastroenterology*, **55**, 522–544.

MEINHARD, E., McRAE, C. U. & CHISHOLM, G. D. (1973). Testicular biopsy in the evaluation of male infertility. *Brit. med. J.*, **iii**, 577–581.

SCHEUER, P. J. (1973). *Liver Biopsy Interpretation*, 2nd edition. London: Baillière, Tindall & Cassell.

Fixation and Fixatives

At the present time no ideal fixative exists, and all solutions have serious drawbacks (i.e. causing tissue shrinkage, slow penetration, etc). It is not our intention to discuss the theory or the effects of fixation, as this is well documented elsewhere, but to describe briefly the purpose of fixation, and to recommend a few of the many fixatives and their application to various staining methods.

Purpose of fixation
1. To preserve the tissue (inhibit autolysis, etc.)
2. To prevent diffusion.
3. To harden the tissue (to facilitate handling and sectioning).
4. To protect the tissue from subsequent treatment (i.e. dehydration).
5. To aid staining reactions.

Consideration to be given to choice of fixative
1. Preservation of cellular detail (e.g. glutaraldehyde gives excellent preservation and is therefore extensively used in electron microscopy).
2. Rate of penetration (e.g. formalin penetrates rapidly; glutaraldehyde and Bouin's fluid penetrate poorly).
3. Amount of shrinkage or swelling. (e.g. Carnoy's fixative gives severe shrinkage).
4. Staining methods to be used (e.g. formol sublimate facilities trichrome staining methods).

FIXATIVE SOLUTIONS

Most of the commonly used fixatives are based on formaldehyde, a simple saturated aliphatic aldehyde. Fixatives utilising formaldehyde alone penetrate tissues well and cause little shrinkage or hardening.

Formaldehyde is the main component of fixatives and is supplied as a saturated solution of formaldehyde gas in water in strengths ranging from 36 to 40 per cent. Confusion can occur over the strength of formaldehyde: 10 per cent formol saline consists of 10 ml of the 40 per cent solution in a total volume of 100 ml. When supplied, formaldehyde is acid, or becomes so on storage due to the formation of formic acid. For its use in histology, formalin should always be brought to neutral pH with suitable buffer solutions; failure to do so will produce formalin pigment (see Chap. 8). Formaldehyde is an irritant to the respiratory epithelium and also to the eyes. It should never be used in a closed space, or added to hot water.

Formalin fixes proteins by complex crosslinking; it does not fix lipids but preserves them well, especially when used with calcium ions.

Formol saline

This fixative, which is generally used as 10 per cent solution of formaldehyde in normal saline, is the most widely used of all fixatives and is recommended for the demonstration of lipids and cell nuclei. It is the best primary fixative available, allowing suitable secondary fixation to be employed before using acid dyes, as in the van Gieson or trichrome stains. As discussed in Chapter 8, unbuffered formalin fixatives can produce a brown pigment when used as an acid solution and in contact with blood-containing tissues.

There are two drawbacks to this fixative. It is not ideal for very urgent biopsy work, since faster penetration and fixation can be obtained with other fixatives e.g. Carnoy's fixative. In addition, formol saline does not protect the tissue well from subsequent shrinkage during dehydration with alcohols (although formol saline itself causes very little shrinkage during the fixation process).

Formol sublimate

This fixative, used as a 10 per cent solution of formaldehyde in saturated aqueous mercuric chloride, is an excellent fixative for the routine surgical laboratory. It considerably enhances the staining of acid dyes and is recommended for trichrome methods and cytoplasmic stains generally. However, silver methods do not give the best possible results with this fixative. The fixative produces a mercury precipitate which can be removed by treatment with iodine, followed by alcohol or sodium thiosulphate.

Zenker's fixative

This solution contains mercuric chloride, potassium dichromate, sodium sulphate and acetic acid, and produces good connective tissue stains. In our hands it has no advantage over formol sublimate. It produces good results with bone marrow biopsies if the tissue is freshly fixed. It hardens tissue more than formol sublimate and also produces the mercury deposit.

Helly's fixative

This fixative has the same contents as Zenker's with the substitution of formalin for the acetic acid. It allows better nuclear staining than Zenker's, whilst being excellent for connective tissue stains and marrow biopsies. It does produce considerable tissue hardening and is not suitable for routine use.

Carnoy's fixative

This fluid, which contains absolute alcohol, chloroform and acetic acid in the proportion of 6:3:1, is recommended as a rapid fixative for urgent biopsy material. Tissue blocks 3 mm thick are fixed within one hour. Blocks are transferred direct from Carnoy's fixative to absolute alcohol before being cleared. It is of no value for long fixation since with fixation times over one hour it produces severe shrinkage.

Bouin's fixative

This gives excellent results with connective tissue stains, particularly, in our experience, with the MSB method of Lendrum et al (1962) although the original authors recommend formol sublimate. It is generally a good routine fixative, and is particularly useful for the fixation of renal biopsy cores, since

K

the Jones methenamine silver method gives excellent results with a reduced silver incubation time using this fixative. However, good fixation of wedge biopsies is not obtained with this fixative as penetration is slow.

Formol calcium
A good all round fixative, especially recommended for lipids and histochemical methods when a fixative is required. It is used at 4°C.

VAPOUR FIXATION
A number of chemicals can be used to fix tissues by the vapours they emit. This type of fixation has long been used to fix smears and sections. The main advantage of vapour fixation is in the fixation of soluble substances; these are often rendered insoluble after vapour fixation but are washed out in liquid fixatives. Vapour fixation is also used with freeze-dried tissue. Formaldehyde gas is the most widely used vapour fixative.

Routine formaldehyde vapour fixation
A small piece of cotton wool soaked in concentrated formaldehyde solution is packed into the bottom of a suitable container, e.g. Coplin jar, and the slides bearing the sections or smears to be fixed are inserted upright. Time for adequate fixation depends upon the thickness of the smear or section.

Formaldehyde vapour fixation of freeze-dried tissue
Freeze-dried tissue is often fixed in formaldehyde vapour. It is essential that the tissue is kept as dry as possible, so the formaldehyde vapour used is generated by heating paraformaldehyde powder at 50–80°C; this process is continued for 2–3 hours, by which time fixation should be complete.

FIXATIVES FOR 1μ SECTIONS AND ELECTRON MICROSCOPY
Glutaraldehyde
This aldehyde solution was introduced as a primary fixative for electron microscopy in the early 1960s. It is a fast-acting aldehyde which produces excellent preservation of cellular detail. Although fast-acting, it has a slow rate of penetration and it is only suitable for use with small pieces of tissue. For electron microscopy it is usually followed by secondary fixation with osmium tetroxide. Glutaraldehyde is used in a buffered solution, using a phosphate or cacodylate buffer; these also increase the osmolarity of the fixative solution and improve the results obtained.

Since glutaraldehyde gives such excellent preservation it is also the fixative of choice for 1μ toluidine blue stained sections.

Osmium tetroxide
Osmium tetroxide is used as a 1 per cent buffered solution. It has fallen out of favour as a primary fixative but is used as a secondary fixative after glutaraldehyde fixation since it preserves lipoprotein membranes better than glutaraldehyde. An additional advantage is that osmium tetroxide is electron-dense and therefore gives good contrast on electron microscopy.

Paraformaldehyde

This is a useful compromise fixative when the ultimate fate of a piece of tissue is not known, i.e. whether it is to be used for subsequent araldite embedding and electron microscopy or whether it is to be processed in a routine manner for paraffin embedding. When paraformaldehyde is used within about four hours of its preparation it is a suitable fixative for electron microscopy; after this time it is little better than ordinary formalin as regards cellular preservation.

FORMULATION OF SOME COMMON FIXATIVE SOLUTIONS

10 per cent formol saline

Formaldehyde	100 ml
Sodium chloride	9 g
Tap water	900 ml

10 per cent formol calcium

Formaldehyde	10 ml
Tap water	90 ml
Calcium chloride	1 g

Lillie's AAF

Formaldehyde	10 ml
Glacial acetic acid (concentrated)	5 ml
Absolute alcohol	85 ml

Gendre's fixative

Saturated picric acid in 95 per cent alcohol	80 ml
Formaldehyde	15 ml
Glacial acetic acid	5 ml

Formol sublimate

Mercuric chloride (saturated aqueous)	90 ml
Formaldehyde	10 ml

Carnoy's fixative

Absolute alcohol	60 ml
Chloroform	30 ml
Glacial acetic acid (concentrated)	10 ml

Bouin's fixative

Picric acid (saturated aqueous)	75 ml
Formaldehyde	25 ml
Glacial acetic acid	5 ml

Zenker's fixative

Mercuric chloride	5 g
Potassium dichromate	2.5 g
Sodium sulphate	1 g
Distilled water	100 ml
Glacial acetic acid (add just before use)	5 ml

Helly's fixative

As above, except 5 ml formaldehyde replaces 5 ml acetic acid.

Paraformaldehyde fixative

Dissolve paraformaldehyde in distilled water to make a 40 per cent solution by heating in a fume cupboard, stirring constantly until only a faint cloudiness persists. Clarify this solution by adding 10N NaOH drop by drop until the solution is clear. Cool to room temperature and then to 4°C in a refrigerator. Filter after cooling to 4°C. If the solution is being used only for subsequent paraffin sections, the longevity of the 40 per cent paraformaldehyde can be increased by adding sodium pyrophosphate until the solution is a 0.02M solution of sodium pyrophosphate in the 40 per cent paraformaldehyde solution.

For electron microscopy. As soon as the 40 per cent paraformaldehyde solution has been cooled and filtered, the working fixative can be prepared:

40 per cent paraformaldehyde solution (as prepared above)	10 ml
0.2M sodium cacodylate buffer (previously adjusted to pH 7.4 with HCl)	45 ml
Distilled water	45 ml

After mixing the three solutions, readjust pH to 7.4 with HCl. Store in a refrigerator at 4°C. Use within 4 hours.

APPENDIX 2
Some Useful Solutions

Acid alcohol

Hydrochloric acid (concentrated)	1 ml
70 per cent alcohol	99 ml

Glycerin jelly
  (a) For use with oxidative enzymes:

Gelatine	15 g
Distilled water	100 ml
Glycerol	100 ml

Slowly dissolve the gelatine in distilled water with moderate heat; when dissolved add the glycerol and mix well. Filter through glass wool whilst hot.

  (b) For general use:

Gelatine	15 g
Distilled water	· 90 ml
Glycerol	105 ml
Phenol crystals	0.5 g

Prepare as in (a) above.

Apathy's mountant (modified by Lillie)

Gum arabic crystals	50 g
Cane sugar	50 g
Distilled water	100 ml
Thymol	100 mg

Dissolve with moderate heating.

Gram's iodine

Iodine	1 g
Potassium iodide	2 g
Distilled water	300 ml

Lugol's iodine

Iodine	1 g
Potassium iodide	2 g
Distilled water	100 ml

Tincture of iodine

Iodine	2 g
Potassium iodide	2 g
Distilled water	2 ml
90 per cent alcohol	74 ml

Gum sucrose

Gum acacia	2 g
Sucrose	60 g
Distilled water	200 ml

Gelatine formaldehyde mixture (for coating slides and coverslips)

1 per cent gelatine	5 ml
2 per cent formaldehyde	5 ml

Coat the slides or coverslips with the above solution; allow to dry before picking up sections.

Definitions

Here are defined, and simply explained, a few of the technical terms which may be unfamiliar to the trainee pathologist, and a few important pathological terms which appear in this book and which may be unfamiliar to technologists. It is in no way a full glossary of the terms used in histopathology.

ACID DYE: These dyes usually stain tissue cytoplasm. They have a reactive acid component and a neutral base. An example is eosin.

ANAPLASTIC: see 'Poorly differentiated'.

ARGYROPHILIA: this term broadly means having an affinity for silver. Tissues (e.g. basement membranes), pigments (e.g. melanin) and micro-organisms (e.g. fungi) which can be stained by the deposition of silver are said to be *argyrophilic*. Note that the word argyrophil is sometimes used in a rather more specific sense when applied to certain types of specialised epithelial cells (see Chap. 8).

ATROPHY: a word used to describe a reduction in size of an organ, tissue or cells, usually associated with a reduction in function. Many factors can cause atrophy, e.g. the brain atrophies in old age, probably because of a very gradual reduction in arterial blood supply; the uterus atrophies after the menopause because its hormonal stimulus slowly reduces.

AUTOFLUORESCENCE: is the ability of tissues to exhibit fluorescence *without* any pretreatment when viewed with a fluorescence microscope.

BASIC DYES: these dyes will stain cell nuclei. They have a reactive base component in combination with non-reactive acid. An example is haematoxylin.

BIREFRINGENCE: see 'Polarisation'.

BLUEING: is a term applied to the treatment of haematoxylin-stained sections by alkaline solutions, usually tap water. This is necessary because the most intense coloration of haematoxylin occurs in alkaline solutions. After differentiation with acid alcohol, haematoxylin-stained structures appear pale. Treatment with alkaline solutions increases the intensity of staining. Even without differentiation the blueing process is essential because most haematoxylin solutions are prepared as acid solutions.

CHELATING AGENT: is an organic chemical which is capable of strongly combining with metals, e.g. ethylenediamine tetra-acetic acid combines strongly with calcium, and is used in decalcification.

DICHROISM: (see first 'Polarisation') is the effect obtained with amyloid fibrils and Congo red. Amyloid unstained is weakly birefringent. When stained with Congo red it becomes strongly birefringent and *dichroic*, that is to say, as well as appearing bright against a dark background, when the specimen is orientated to obtain maximum intensity the colour of the birefringence will change from yellow to green.

DYSPLASIA: a descriptive term applied to an epithelium which shows abnormalities of size, shape and nuclear content of its constituent cells. A dysplastic epithelium is in a state of unrest, and dysplasia is a danger signal, warning of possible subsequent malignant change in the epithelium.

FLUOROCHROME: is a dye which will exhibit fluorescence when viewed under the fluorescent microscope. It is usually capable of reasonably specific binding to certain tissue structures, e.g. thioflavine T to demonstrate amyloid.

HETEROTOPIC: means 'out of place'. Heterotopic calcification is the name given to calcification which occurs where it is not normally found, e.g. in the kidney.

INFARCT: an area of tissue death brought about by an interference with the blood supply of the area, usually an abrupt impairment of its arterial supply.

METACHROMASIA: is the ability of a few basic dyes to stain certain tissue components a colour different from the colour of the dye itself. An example is toluidine blue which stains acid mucosubstances red.

MORDANT: a mordant is a substance which forms a link between, and has a strong affinity for, a dye and a tissue structure. The mordant is usually a metal, e.g. aluminium which is used with haematoxylin. The linkage between the dye and the tissue is called a dye-lake.

NECROSIS: means tissue death. It can be caused by many factors, including loss of blood supply (see 'Infarction' above), infection by microorganisms, trauma, etc.

ORTHOCHROMASIA: is the colour obtained with a metachromatic dye, that is the same colour as the dye itself, e.g. blue with toluidine blue.

POLARISATION: is a technique used in the examination of cells and tissues. It gives information about the existence of preferentially orientated constituents and the direction of their orientation. A polarising microscope has a Nicol prism or, if a modified microscope, a polaroid disc below the condenser and an analyser or polaroid disc between the specimen stage and the eyepieces. When the planes of polarisation of polariser and analyser are perpendicular no light passes through the ocular. If a specimen is examined under these conditions orientated constituents may become visible on a dark field. The intensity will be maximum when the specimen is viewed at 45° to the planes of polarisation of polariser and analyser. Objects having internal regularity of structure may have two descriptive refractive indices, hence showing *birefringence*. The structure of amyloid is regular enough to show this effect, which is enhanced with selective Congo red staining.

POORLY DIFFERENTIATED: when the cells of which a tumour is composed do not closely resemble the cell of origin, but have sufficient characteristic features remaining to enable the cell type to be identified, the tumour is said to be poorly differentiated. When the tumour cells are so poorly differentiated that it is not possible to identify the cell type, the tumour is said to be *anaplastic*. (cf 'Well differentiated').

PROGRESSIVE STAINING: is when the tissue is stained to the correct intensity with the dye; it is usually used when the dye has an affinity for a specific tissue structure.

PYRAMITOME: is a microtome for trimming resin-embedded blocks before sectioning for the electron microscope. It can also be used to produce $1\,\mu$ thick resin-embedded sections for the light microscope. It uses a glass knife.

REGRESSIVE STAINING: is the overstaining of sections with a dye and the selective removal of the dye in a differentiator. Alum haematoxylin as a dye and acid alcohol as a differentiator are good examples.

SECONDARY FIXATION: is the process of employing a second fixative to tissue fixed or partially fixed, usually in formaldehyde. The secondary fixative is often formal mercuric chloride. It is often used to enhance some staining methods, e.g. the trichrome stains.

ULTRAMICROTOME: a sophisticated microtome using a glass or diamond knife to cut sections of resin-embedded material suitable for use with an electron microscope, i.e. approximately 40 nm (400 Å) thick.

WELL DIFFERENTIATED: when the cells of which a tumour is composed closely resemble the cell of origin, the tumour is said to be well differentiated (cf 'Poorly differentiated').

Index

Note: page numbers in **bold type** indicate the location of the practical method.

Printed by
THOMSON LITHO LTD., EAST KILBRIDE, SCOTLAND

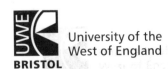